MW01058040

Fitness Hacks:
Cheat Your Way to a Better Body Today!

"Tricks and Tactics for More Motivation, Less Fat and an Awesome Body Fast!"

Phil Pierce

Copyright © 2014

www.BlackBeltFit.com

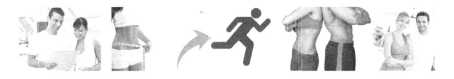

What Can You Get From This Book?

- Do you know how to slash your workout time to 4 minutes AND get better results, with one tactic?

- Want to learn how you can burn calories even if you like watching TV or playing video games all day?

- Discover how to unlock your brain with proven psychological hacks

- How one simple change can give you all-day unstoppable energy

- The incredible truth about weight loss that you NEED to hear!

- Why you can afford to skip _____ but never _____

- How to trick your mind into eating less, even if you hate diets!

- Secret tips for hacking your gym

- The one easy change to your daily routine that burns thousands of calories!

- How to avoid the biggest gym mistake 90% of people make

- Revealed: the biggest hidden obstacle to weight loss, and how to destroy it.

- Quick tips and tricks to boost your body and mind

And more!

Do you want to skip the grind and 'cheat' your way to a better body today?

Fitness Hacks reveals the powerful secret tips and tricks YOU can easily use in your daily life to lose weight, build muscle or get fit fast even if you've no motivation, time or money! This expert guide, with insights from top instructors, fitness coaches and cutting-edge research, skips the BS and hard work and exposes the efficiency shortcuts you can take right now to improve your body today!

In fact many of the tactics included will have you getting fit without even knowing it!

With over 50 effective and intelligent Tips and Tricks for your Home, Gym, Exercise, Diet and Mind this guide contains the latest information to help you quickly and efficiently sculpt the body you want. Discover a new way to get in shape today with Fitness Hacks.

Contents

What Can You Get From This Book? 2

Free Bonus Book! 7

Foreword: Hacks vs. Cheats 8

Hacking Your Daily Routine and Making it Stick 10

Foreword: From the Author 12

Bonus: Bestselling Amazon Fitness Author Derek Doepker Gives his No.1 Trick For Instant Motivation! 14

Exercise Hacks: 19

1. Why You Can Save Time Right Now and Skip the... 20

2. But Never Skip the... 23

3. Do it First 27

4. 10% for Lifelong Results 29

5. How to Listen to Your Body 31

6. Choose Your Tunes for Increased Endurance 34

7. Your Extra Set Challenge 37

8. The Power of Supersets! 39

9. How to Get Incredible Results in Minutes! (Not hours) 42

10. Start Drinking 45

Gym Hacks: 48

1. Get Through the Door 49

2. Upgrade to a Nicer Gym 52

3. Use Your Boss 55

4. Hack Your Gym Fees Down 57

5.   Use the Buddy System 60

6.   How to Avoid the No.1 Weight Mistake 62

7.   New Clothes: New Motivation 65

8.   Get Paid for Working Out! 67

9.   Listen To a Story 70

10.   Look at Yourself 72

Hacks At Home: 74

1.   Skip the Gym (Wait, what?)...................................75

2.   Play Video Games to Get Fit 78

3.   Watch Television 81

4.   Share Online...................................84

5.   How One Change to Your Workspace Can Burn Thousands of Calories! 86

6.   Supercharge Your Walk 90

7.   Brush Your Teeth and Build Muscle 93

8.   The No.1 Tactic for Beating Stress 95

9.   Trick Your Brain Into Eating Less With… 97

10.   How to Clean Up Your Act 99

Cheating While Eating (Diet Hacks): 101

1.   Go Bananas! 102

2.   Cheating Your Way To 5-A-Day...................................104

3.   How to 'Top-Load' Your Day for Unstoppable Energy 108

4.   When to Fuel Up Before Your Workout...................................112

5.   Take Emotional Eating to the Curb 115

6.   Organize Your Refrigerator.............................117

7.   Brilliant Beta Glucans.................................119

8.   Choosing Superfoods...................................121

9.   The Great Vitamin Myth................................132

10.   The Shocking Truth About Diets! 134

Mind Hacks: 138

1.   Calendar Crosses for Unbeatable Habits 139

2.   The Right Words For You...............................141

3.   How to Physically Improve Your Brain - Learn How to
Meditate in just 2 Minutes! 144

4.   Why You Should Ditch Weigh-Ins and BMI B.S. 148

5.   Turn Reps on Their Head to Make Exercise Easier.....152

6.   Hack Your Sleep, Recharge Your Mind (and Body).....154

7.   Why You Should Forget Weight Loss (For Now) 158

8.   Run...for Survival! 160

9.   Live In the Now and Destroy Mental Resistance 162

10.   The One Incredible Thing You Can Do Right Now to
Feel Instantly Happier.....................................164

Bonus Quick Tips 166

Thank You (and a Free Book!) 168

Other Books by Phil Pierce...............................169

Free Bonus Book!

Grab your Completely Free bonus book;
'How to Develop Power with Plyometrics' now!

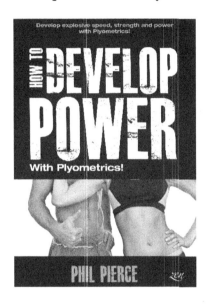

Just head over to my site:

Claim your copy now!

Foreword: Hacks vs. Cheats

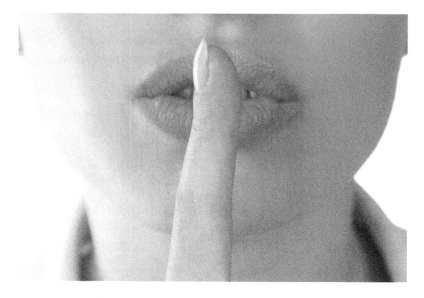

It's important to understand that the advice in this guide is not deception or trickery but your insight to shortcuts for real long term health improvements. There are no smoke and mirrors and no 'cheats' in the most literal sense.

The advice included within this book is centered on helping you become ruthlessly efficient in improving your body by skipping the pointless hard work or the confusing myths and giving you the lifestyle tips with the most return for your time and effort, all backed up by the latest research and innovations in health and fitness.

Some of the techniques in this guide are quick tips, others are clever changes you can make to your daily routine for longer term health benefits but in each case they are focused on easy methods for self-improvement.

Why take the long route if you can skip straight to the bit you need?

Efficiency is the name of the game here and maximizing every spare moment to get fit, often without even realising it!

This book is not for everyone though and not every tip will be relevant to you, but even if only one of them strikes a chord (and I guarantee a few will) then you will go forward with the powerful knowledge to improve your body while saving time, money and stress for the rest of your life.

You don't have to rush out and use all of these tactics. In fact I wouldn't recommend trying to introduce more than a few at a time but knowledge is power in the fitness game and even just knowing one or two simple adjustments to your life can have long term benefits.

This book is all about the easy wins, the sneaky tactics and the hidden tricks to get you in amazing shape in record time!

Let's get started! ...

Hacking Your Daily Routine and Making it Stick

Would you like to improve your body AND make it last?

You'll see the term 'mental resistance' (and ways to beat it) come up several times in this book. In summary it is the conscious push-back we have in our mind when we think about something difficult, tiring or perceived to be hard work.

It's for this very reason that the many lifestyle changes promoted by the myriad diets, self-help gurus and other experts simply won't stick in the long term. They are easy to read about, easy to get excited about in some book or website, but once we examine the process further we realise it requires huge adjustments to our daily life.

In general we like our life the way it is; our brain craves stability and doesn't want this to change. When thoughts of a big alterations to our daily existence enter our mind they becomes an obstacle we simply can't overcome. It builds and builds until we discard it altogether.

It's for this reason that this guide takes a completely different approach.
Yes this book can change your life and massively improve your health, but not by making you undergo drastic changes or forcing you to face pain and suffering.

This book focuses on "easy wins". The effective and fast lifestyle changes so simple that you barely even consider them, and ultimately find it easy to introduce them as part of a regular routine.

Consider driving a car. If you drive over a large rock in the road you will stop to get out and examine it, probably stress about it and the journey will be interrupted. But if you drive over a pebble, or even a series or pebbles they are barely noticeable, not even worth worrying about.

This book helps keep you on your fitness journey.

Routine is key

Or to put it another way, 'systems' are key. Whether you are trying to lose weight, improve motivation or just have vague ideas of getting healthy, establishing an easy to follow system that integrates smoothly and with little-to-no mental resistance is the only way it will stick.

That isn't to say you should start developing a database or filling your calendar with notes and schedules (although that works for some). More that by setting up regularity with your activities your mind will find it much easier to deal with the actions and establish a base for your fitter life.

Create a simple schedule for your changes and start small. Once you successfully introduce one to your life move onto the next and so on. After a short time you will have established a solid fitness foundation for the rest of your life.

Foreword: From the Author

Face it, you are lazy.

Don't worry I am too.

In fact so is everyone else.

It's not that we can't be bothered to get up off the couch (although for some people that can be the case!); it's that as a species humanity has developed the ability to seek the shortest possible path to a goal. We have the brain power to see all the various routes to what we wish to achieve and deduce the most efficient and economical method of attaining them.

Be that getting to a destination, finding food to eat or learning a topic. We simply jump in the car, head to the microwave or look online for what we want.

Despite how it may seem, on an intellectual level this is actually a beautiful thing. In evolutionary terms for example this has led to most of the modern technology we take for granted and the advancement of the human race. (Where would we be without the invention of the wheel, or time saving devices like cars and telephones)?

But the downside of this school of thought is that, in the modern, energy saving world, we really have less reason to get active. Whereas in ye-olde days we would have to work hard for our food, our family and to outrun dangers, in the modern world there are no such threats and no primal motivation forcing us to run, jump and climb.

So to get in shape we can either force ourselves to endure the unwanted hard work and mental struggle, ultimately leading to poor motivation and performance or we can use shortcuts to get in shape the easy way!

Imagine your fitness as a destination. There are lots of distractions and different routes to take to get there but with the right information you can ignore the myths and unnecessary hard work and take the most direct route to your goal.

The idea behind this guide is to use this principle of physical and mental efficiency for our own gain. To use the cheats and shortcuts we so desperately crave to improve our body and enhance our health. Best of all these are all healthy, effective and safe techniques that can drastically improve your life!

So here is a guide for all you economists out there. For all you people who want fitness results without the pointless time wasting!

Fitness Hacks is your shortcut to a better body today.

- *Phil*

Bonus: Bestselling Amazon Fitness Author Derek Doepker Gives his No.1 Trick For Instant Motivation!

As a friend, fitness expert and bestselling author I asked Derek Doepker to offer his own special insights into fitness and well-being...

Henry Ford says "whether you believe you can or can't, you're right." One of the biggest roadblocks to fitness success that I've seen in both myself and others are the limiting beliefs someone can tell themselves like "I don't have enough time" "I don't have enough money" "I can't stop myself from eating junk food" "I hate exercise" etc.

When a person tells themselves these things, their brain will literally not let them see any other alternative. And I've found it doesn't really do someone any good to tell some "just think positively" without showing them how to actually go inside their brain and change their beliefs.

The technique I'm going to share with you is my #1 technique to overcome excuses, unlock creative problem solving abilities, and will ideally be used in every area of your life you want to improve. If you took this piece of advice and ran with it, I believe it could be *the* answer to everything that you feel is holding you back. That's not an exaggeration. This technique is what changed every area of my life, not just my health.

Before I understood how the brain worked, I would often tell myself things like "I hate healthy food and I can't give up my favorite fast food meals." Then I realized that these sorts of beliefs are created and reinforced by the language that runs through the mind, often subconsciously.

Each day we tell and ask ourselves all sorts of things. These things could be "I don't have enough time." "I'm a failure." "Why can't I overcome my junk food cravings?"

or alternatively...
"I can make time to exercise twice this week" "I am successful" "What do I love about eating healthy foods?"

The one thing I've found can turn everything around is simply changing one's language patterns from dis-empowering statements and dis-empowering questions to instead asking high quality questions.

One reason this technique works is because I can't tell you what will work best for your life. Instead, the best answers and solutions for you will always come from within yourself, even if it takes the help of someone else to draw it out of you.

Here's an experiment. Try saying these things to yourself and see how you feel:
"I don't know what to do."
"Everything is hopeless."
"Why is there never enough time?"
"What is wrong with me?

Be honest with yourself, even if you haven't ever made these exact statements in your own life, have you ever told or asked yourself something that made things seem impossible or extremely difficult? Have these things ever at times been things that you really knew weren't totally true?

Let's replace these with "empowering questions." See how you feel when asking these things:

"What's one simple thing that I can do right now to start moving me forward even more?"
"What can I do with the time I do have?"
"What healthier foods do I enjoy?"
"How can I make healthier foods taste even better?"
"Why am I getting even more fit each day?"
"How can I make getting fit even more enjoyable?"
"How can I do the best that I can?"

Now, as a tip, try asking questions that can improve your outlook on life in general like:

"When have I been successful in the past?"
"How does it get even better than this?"
"Why is everything working out for the best even if I can't see it?"

Let's take the sample question: "What's one simple thing that I can do right now to start moving me forward even more?"

The answer doesn't have to be something big. Maybe it's just doing 5 jumping jacks in the morning or replacing a candy bar with a piece of fruit.

Then keep asking the question regularly and build up more and more. They would ask "could I do 10 jumping jacks a day and add in 10 pushups?" If the answer is yes, they do that.

When that is comfortable, they ask themselves "could I go even further?"
Not all questions will have an answer right away. Let's say you ask "how can I make exercise extremely fun?" and you don't come up with an answer. Some questions will either not have a clear answer, or will be too outside of your current knowledge zone for you to determine a solution.

Then try another question like "how can I make exercise at least a little more enjoyable?"

Perhaps that's by listening to an audio book while exercising or setting up a friendly competition with others with prizes for whoever makes the most progress in their exercise routine. The great thing is, whatever answer you come up with will be your own.

The point of this is not that asking one question will solve all your problems just like one workout won't get you a dream body. It's the consistent practice and making it a habit that will change your life.

Thomas Edison failed over 1000 times when creating the light bulb. The reason he succeeded is because inventors are naturally curious.

He said that each failure was a success in getting closer to finding a solution. Rather than saying "I messed up, I'm a failure." Or asking "why do I never succeed?" He may have asked "given that this didn't work, what can I do differently that will move me closer to creating this light bulb?" "What do I need to learn or try to make this work?" Etc.

What you focus on expands!
If that's problems, you'll see more problems. If that's potential solutions to problems, you'll start to see more solutions. Not always right away, but eventually the brain will start to see new things and make connections that you could have never thought of before.

Here's another example:
"What's one healthier food I can enjoy, afford, and have time to eat?"

Perhaps that's just eating one apple a day. If that's all you can do to change your diet for the next month, that's great! Even if one still eats a bunch of junk food, the point is not to get the perfect diet overnight. It's to be in the practice of constant forward motion and growth so that, a year later, one has made a noticeable difference. (It will likely happen much sooner though!)

No matter how seemingly insignificant the step forward is, it will start to snowball. This is more about changing psychology and language patterns than it is one's physical body at first. Apply this to every area of your life, and it will be impossible for it not to change for the better.

Use your own questions and you'll discover your own answers.

This advice is worth more than gold if you truly apply it to your life. If struggling to find a good question, you can always ask yourself "what's a good question to ask?"

In all my years of studying health, psychology, and personal development, I've found this simple insight: The answer is a question.

- Derek

Want More Cutting Edge Fitness Tips?

Derek Doepker is the founder of http://excuseproof.com and author of the #1 bestselling book 50 Fitness Tips You Wish You Knew http://amzn.to/U33zCM (Kindle) http://amzn.to/Wn4Ulx (Print)

Exercise Hacks:

Fitness is essentially an instinctive bodily reaction to exercise. When we push our body into activity the muscles, circulatory system and brain reacts to this stimulus and get us ready for action. Do this enough times and the body starts to adapt, building bigger muscles, reducing excess fat and increasing tolerance to the hard work.

As the body gets better at handling hard work so do we find we are healthier and leaner. Our mental state of mind also improves as exercise releases endorphins and happy-inducing hormones. The brain tells the body that running around and getting out of breath is good!

All-in-all exercise triggers very positive physical and mental changes, programmed by nature to make us enjoy being as active in the way our bodies were designed for.

So why is it such an unappealing prospect for many people?

Most people think of exercise as hours of slogging away at the gym or sweating on a treadmill but this doesn't have to be the way. In fact that approach is probably just wasting your time when you can get the same results in minutes. (More on that to come…)

The aim of the following tips and tactics is to cut through the fog of misinformation and give you a more direct route to powerful results making your exercise sessions easier, quicker and more efficient than ever before.

1. Why You Can Save Time Right Now and Skip the…

…Stretching.

Warming up is crucial but recent discoveries show that stretching, well, isn't.

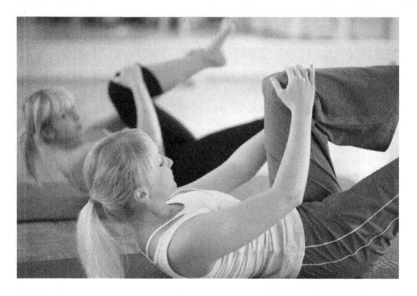

- "Skip the old static (Muscle-pulling) stretches and you can <u>increase</u> your power!"

I discuss this topic and more in my book "How to Stretch for Martial Arts and Fitness" (http://bit.ly/1dhkYUk) but essentially static, old school-style stretching, is probably just wasting your time.

Whereas in the old days, recommendations for effectiveness were often based on anecdotes and hearsay from surly old 'experts', today we have the hard facts and figures backing up the claims, and revealing some surprising truths.

Experts in the field of kinesiology are now publishing strongly documented reports that indicate much of what we take for granted when training is actually outright wrong!

You see most of us have been doing the same type of limbering up since school. We'd stand in a freezing field pulling our legs left and right while a sadistic gym instructor prepared to force us on a freezing 6 mile run. (Well, that was my school experience anyway).

It turns out however that static stretches, the type where you stand and slowly pull a limb until you meet resistance, is not only useless in warming up the muscles but actually reduces the strength of that muscle's output for a short time afterwards.

A recent study carried out by the University of Nevada revealed that athletes produced less force from leg muscles after doing a series of static (traditional) stretches, than if they had done no stretching at all!

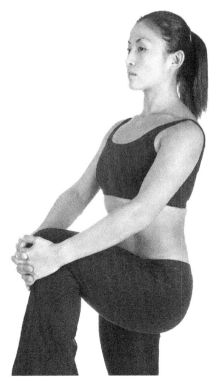

Other research has shown up to a 30 percent decrease in muscle strength after static stretching and that static stretches can even affect other limbs. (In theory due to the impact on the central nervous system as a whole).

Shocking Stuff.

A "neuromuscular inhibitory response" is the culprit; effectively your body and muscles reacting negatively and resisting the static stretch. While you might feel more flexible initially, the actual muscular output is lessened and you've simply increased mental tolerance to the sensation.

Instead all studies now point to Dynamic Stretching and Dynamic Warm Ups as the optimal way to prepare for activity.

Dynamic Stretching/Warm Up:

-   Increases Blood Flow
-   Works full range of motion
-   Increases Power
-   Improves Flexibility

In fact Dynamic Stretches and warm ups were shown in a recent CDC study to cut injury rates by around 50% compared with the alternatives.

2. But Never Skip the…

…Warm Up.

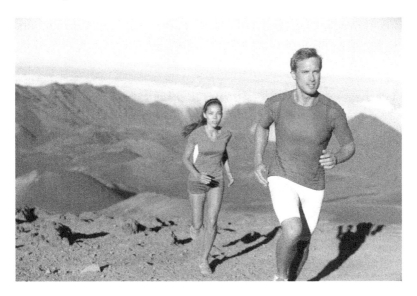

- "Warm up to improve performance and make it easy by doing what you do."

Firstly **always** warm up. If you get the body loose and prepared for movement you greatly reduce the risk of injury and the chances that you may be out of action for an extended spell. Better to spend couple of minutes gently moving around than 3 weeks out with a torn muscle!

Secondly, and perhaps more importantly the simple act of preparing for exercise gets your mind in the right frame for what is to come.

It's funny that so many of us dread exercise. We think of any excuse we can to not do it.

So don't do it. Just warm up instead.

Instead of thinking about some large task to complete like a 5 mile run or 2 hour fitness class just focus on the warm-up and getting your body moving in a gentle manner. By doing this you remove that mental barrier and start the fitness process.

While specific stretches aid in preparing localized muscle groups for action, and reduce stiffness and tension after an event, warming up as a whole is just as important to introduce the body to the activity it is about to undertake.

The latest research and scientific developments may be changing our opinions about traditional stretches and how effective (or wasteful) static stretches really are but interestingly these studies have also revealed the most effective way to warm- up in general for an activity and lucky for us it's very simple;

"Do what you do"

That is, most studies have now shown that the best way to warm up for a specific activity is to do that activity - though at a reduced intensity.

It's not rocket science, and yet for years all sorts of new and trendy pseudo-science approaches to warming up have been adopted in different fitness circles. Thankfully common sense is finally getting the backup it deserves from concrete results and we are now seeing some sensible approaches to warm up exercises that are non-technical and actually good for your body!

Simply put;

If you are a runner, to warm up you need to run.

If you are a swimmer, then swim.

A Martial Artist should make a few kicks and punches. (Depending on your style)

Intensity is Key

There is a slight caveat to this approach though, in that you don't throw yourself into the activity at full strength straight away. That kind of shock to the system does no good for your body. Instead introduce the exercise at a lower intensity, then a slightly higher intensity, then the full speed, normal activity.

For example, a warm up for runners might be;

- 5 minutes walking at a quick pace - 30% of normal running speed
- 5 minutes jogging slightly faster – 50% of normal running speed
- Finally begin to pick up the pace and run at normal speed.

A simple warm up for Martial Artists;

- Light Shadow Boxing/Sparring for 2 mins
- Slightly faster sparring for 2 mins
- Full Normal Speed sparring (with a partner if needed)

The times have been slightly reduced for sparring because it is already a quite intense exercise

This simple approach of "Do what you do" makes it easy to warm up safely and since you already know the activity there are no complicated techniques for you to work out or potentially get wrong.

Your activity at 20-30% intensity (for 5-10 mins)
To
Your activity at 40-50% intensity (for 5-10 mins)
To
Your activity at normal full intensity

Give it a go!

Another top, full-body warm up:

Bear Crawl

There are a number of dynamic exercises but any full body exercise can work well. An increasingly popular example is the "Spider-man" or as it's known in some circles the "Bear-Crawl".

Simply drop to all fours and walk the length of the gym, room or training hall then back again. This engages most of the body and is an excellent all-body dynamic warm up.

3. Do it First

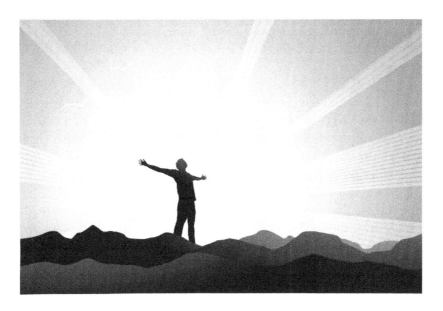

-*"Exercise first thing in the day for improved motivation, sleep and weight management"*

Evidence shows that the morning is the very best time to exercise for several reasons. Sure, it wakes your body up, shakes off any sluggishness from the night before and means you are not tired from work or other activities, but research also indicates that those who exercise in the morning are more likely to stick to it.

Not only that but morning activity was shown in an Appalachian State University investigation to improve the sleep cycle the following night, and a good night's sleep is key to successful weight loss/management.

Best of all a recent study by Brigham Young University also showed early indications that mild morning exercise reduces unwanted snacking by lowering appetite later in the day. Participants showed a lower neural response to food. Perfect if you are trying to lower your sugar intake in the afternoon.

So schedule an early morning workout. By getting it done first, you eliminate the chance that obstacles will appear throughout the day, preventing you from following through with your fitness intentions. Many people intend to workout during their lunch break, or after work, only to find that there is no time left. Be careful not to fall into this fitness pit.

The characteristics which surround the morning also provide greater advantages. If you have windows in your workout space, then you can watch the sunrise during the fall and winter seasons. In summer or hot countries the air will be cooler, allowing you to get active before the temperature really starts to heat up.

Once you are done with your workout, you can shower and get ready for work with the confidence that you began your day doing something great for your body. This will make you more likely to make good choices throughout the day. Working out in the morning will also boost your metabolism for several hours. You will burn more calories throughout the day without any additional exercise.

When you workout first thing in the morning you are more likely to workout consistently. You can even sleep in comfortable workout clothes to ensure that you are ready to begin as soon as you roll out of bed. Once you have completed your workout you will feel energized and ready to take on any challenges that come your way.

4.10% for Lifelong Results

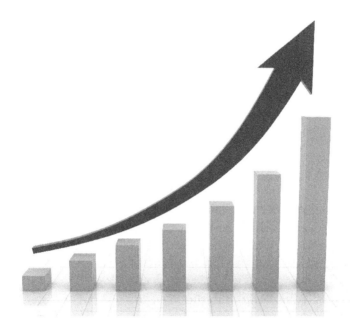

- *"Increase your exercise intensity by 10% at each interval to improve long term motivation and muscle development"*

Did you ever try to learn an instrument or a new language only to see the size of the task ahead and give up? The same applies to fitness. We see the goal and get excited but then we realize just how much work is involved and it seems impossible. This thought then destroys motivation.

Alternatively we throw ourselves into fitness too hard, too fast and get injured, again ruining our best intentions.

It has been proven that gradual progress is most sustainable for long term health. A bite sized approach to getting fit.

Start off small and increase the intensity of your workouts every few sessions to challenge your muscles and encourage progress. It is important to make these changes gradually though. Once you reach a new level in your workout, you can begin planning your next increase.

Progress is essential because if you always do the same one-mile run or thirty-minute stroll three, or four times a week, then your fitness level will plateau. This is because your body becomes accustomed to this level, eliminating the need for increases in your strength or lung capacity.

Instead, make changes gradually, allowing your body the time it needs to get used to each new level of stress. Allow at least two weeks between each addition of increased weight, or duration. Only increase your routine by around **ten percent** or less at any one time. This means that you should not lengthen your run or the number of repetitions you perform by more than ten percent at a time. While this number may be considered conservative in some training circles, it will help you avoid burnout and reduce your risk of exercise related injuries.

By revving up your workout in this way, you will put yourself on the road to optimal lifelong fitness and increase your fat burning capacity for the long haul, not a quick burn-out followed by failure.

Higher intensity fitness programs will eventually help you burn more calories, and improve your overall performance further but to reach them take the ten percent approach and build your body slowly but surely.

5. How to Listen to Your Body

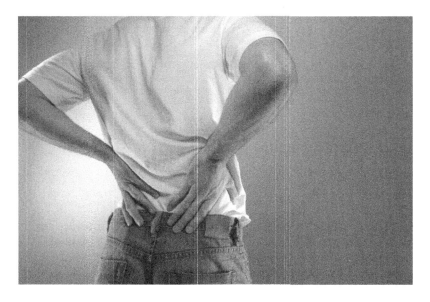

- *"Learn to listen to your body and the difference between 'Pain' and 'Discomfort'"*

Wanting to push yourself is admirable but being able to listen to your body is a skill many overlook.

By paying attention to your body, you will begin to instinctively avoid common exercise related injuries. You can mold a routine, which is both safe and beneficial and remind yourself that staying safe and healthy is more important than speeding up your results.

When you ignore your body's cues, you put yourself at greater risk for injury. By tuning in, you will learn the distinctive difference between normal discomfort and pain. It is vital that you stop any exercise, which produces the sensation of pain. Pain is your body's means for alerting you to a problem. When you sense pain, it is important to reduce the intensity of your workout, or change activities all together. You might also need to give your body a little time to rest and repair itself.

Do not listen to any trainer who tells you to work through the pain. This puts you at a high risk for serious injuries, and even chronic problems throughout your future. However, in many cases it is appropriate to work through discomfort. A small degree of discomfort is often needed to encourage the development of greater strength and cardiovascular capacities.

This kind of discomfort should be limited to fatigued muscles and soreness, primarily in the days immediately following your workout. This discomfort should be limited to your muscles. Immediately discontinue any activity, which causes sharp pain or discomfort in your joints or tendons.

Another factor that can be helpful in identifying the difference between pain and normal discomfort is timing. Pain that begins immediately after you start an exercise is a problem. The discomfort of muscle fatigue will not appear until you near the end of your set. Pain that limits your mobility, or appears only on one side of your body is also means for concern.

If your exercises cause pain, you may not be completing them properly or perhaps you have an old injury that is not fully recovered. Slow down and listen to your body for the sake of avoiding a long-term injury, which may haunt you for the duration of your future. Rest and give your body a chance to recover as needed. Use the cues your body gives you to make adjustments needed to develop a safe workout with better results.

Top Tip: Scoring pain – how to listen to your body

Discomfort is a natural part of physical improvement. Outright pain is not. The old idea of no pain no gain is a fallacy invented by sadistic coaches to push people . This may work psychologically but the body has its limits.

If something hurts consider what grade out of ten you would give it. 1 to 7 is discomfort and common among exercise. You should be able to push past it. 7 to 10 is pain and a signal something is wrong. Listen to your body and do not carry on.

1 2 3 4 5 6 7 8 9 10

Discomfort   **Pain**

6. Choose Your Tunes for Increased Endurance

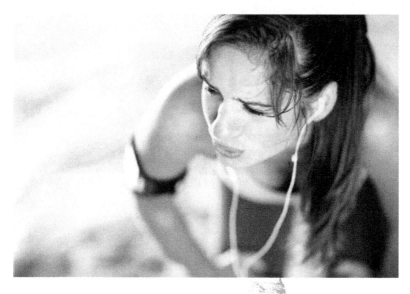

- *"Music is proven to make you work harder for longer and feel less tired. Choose your tunes well!"*

Listening to good music is one of those age-old tricks that really works. In fact it goes all the way back to the early rowers and slaves onboard ancient ships. In those days drummers would beat a rhythm to not only inspire the crew but to establish a pace.

Today studies have shown that "synchronization" with the music (the process of feeling in time) helps you push past mental barriers and endure fatigue.

Collated studies by the University of Wisconsin demonstrated that selecting suitable music lowered perceived exertion in participants during intense cycling, running or other cardio by significant amounts.

This is especially true if you have a habit of constantly glancing at the timer during your cardio or circuit training workouts. Of course, this only serves to make each session seem longer. By creating a playlist that is the same length as your workout, you can remove the clock watching and focus more on your task. In fact, once you stop thinking about how much time you have left, it will seem to fly right by.

This is especially true if you choose songs, which you seriously enjoy. You might even find yourself working out longer just to hear your favorite tune one more time. The intensity of your efforts might also increase as your mind is distracted away from the challenge of each movement.

Do not let your playlist get stale, regularly create new lists or swap with a friend to mix things up. Be sure to seek out a variety of tempos to reduce the boredom inducing predictability that workouts are prone to create. Arrange your songs so that they build up to the quickest tempos and gradually slow for your cool-down session. End your playlist with a soothing song to relax your body and mind. This will also help end your session on a positive note, making you more likely to look forward to your next workout.

In addition to its motivational benefits, new research suggests that listening to music while exercising might boost your mental acuity. If you do not have time to organize, your own playlists there are many great workout sets available. Use your favorite search engine to locate them. Alternatively, you could always just tune your radio to your favorite station.

Listening to music while you exercise is great, but it is still important to put safety first. If you listen to music while you run outside then be sure to keep the volume low enough that you can still hear traffic and any other potential dangers as they approach. A lower volume will also protect your ears from irreversible damage.

Top Tip:

Listening to depressing slow songs is shown to be far less stimulating for activity than up-tempo music, no matter how good the song. (Sorry Radiohead)

Try to stick to **120-140 BPM (Beats per minute)** tunes. Around this tempo you will find a regular upbeat rhythm proven to be more effective and if you are lucky you may find a beat that perfectly matches your exercise or running pattern.

7. Your Extra Set Challenge

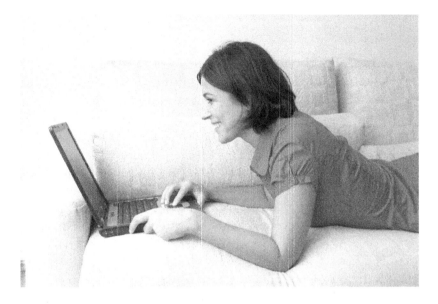

- *"Get some exercise while you check Facebook, watch Youtube or eat snacks with 'Extra Sets'"*

A fun way to fit some bonus exercise in to your day is to require an 'Extra Set' or two of a simple movement before engaging in certain activities.

Are you addicted to checking your e-mail or *facebook*? Do you have a tendency to snack throughout the day?

Make a list of the non-beneficial activities that you tend to do a few times a day such as the ones listed above. Post your list in an obvious place so you are reminded of your promise throughout the day. Alternatively, you can place Post-Its on the objects associated with these actions such as your home computer or refrigerator.

Before engaging any of the habits on your list, choose a basic exercise and complete one or two sets. Jumping jacks, sit-ups, or push-ups are great choices which can be performed anywhere and do not require any equipment.

EG:
- **Check Facebook = 5 Sit Ups**
- **Open Fridge for snack = 5 jumping jacks**
- **Watch a YouTube video = 5 Standing Squats**

Keep the number of reps low to make it manageable and fun.

By the end of the day, you can really stack up some extra repetitions and as we all know when it comes to physical fitness every bit helps. This is especially great if you are looking to improve your fitness level, but do not have time in your schedule to extend your workouts.

Requiring a few sets here and there is also an ideal strategy for beginners. If you are not quite ready to commit yourself to regular workout sessions, you can at least add a little exercise to your day in a fun and painless way. Give it a shot. There is no rule that says you cannot take this one to the office as well although your exercises may have to be adjusted.

An added benefit of this approach is in curing unwanted habits. Say you wish to stop biting your nails. Each time you catch yourself doing this perform a difficult exercise. This will take your mind off the undesired thoughts.

8. The Power of Supersets!

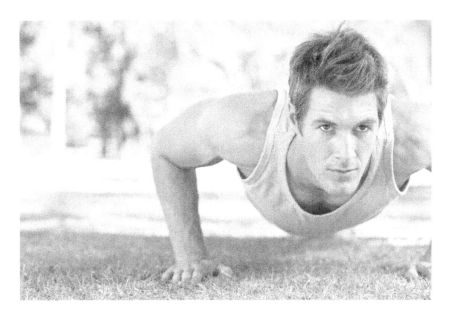

- *"Use 'Supersets' to boost any normal exercise and build muscle faster"*

Supersets are the heroes of the workout world. 'Super' - get it? Ok, that was pretty bad but they are powerful techniques that can help you get results fast.

Complete supersets by performing two exercises but do not stop to pause or rest in between the two sets, essentially linking the movements. To increase the intensity pair two exercises that work the same body region. By repeatedly completing supersets involving a particular group such as your biceps, you can enact the 'overload principle' proven to build muscle. This is a fantastic way to develop strenght without lifting heavy weights.

On the other hand, go for full body results by working opposing regions such as your chest and back. There really are no rules when it comes to Supersets besides pairing exercises with no break. In fact, you can go for body parts that are completely different such as shoulder presses followed by squats. Continue alternating as long as you please.

Example 1: Push up, squat thrusts

A great example of a full body 'Superset' would be a push up, squat thrust combination.

As the push-up finishes you are already in the perfect position to complete a squat thrust. Try 10 Push-up/Squat Thrust combinations or try 10 push-ups then go straight into 10 Squat thrusts.

The advantage here is that you don't need to get up in between each set.

- **Supersets save time by intensifying the exercise**
- **Create muscle growth through overloading**
- **Mix up your routine, preventing boredom**
- **Easily adaptable for intensity**

The point of supersets is to complete a greater amount of work in a small amount of time. This increases both the quality and the intensity of your training session. They also add more convenience to your routine. If you do not have the time for your full workout, you can at least sneak in a superset or two. Alternatively, use supersets throughout your entire session to save time and help your bodywork more efficiently.

You can also make use of supersets when it is time to increase the intensity of your workout. Every few weeks you should change it up to inspire constant improvements. Supersets are a great tool, which allow you to jack up your workout without creating a completely new routine. Judicious use of supersets will keep your workout fun, interesting, and challenging.

Use supersets to spice up your workout. To get started right away, simply pick any two exercises and have at it. Complete a full set of one repeated by a full set of the other. Take a very small rest (or none) and repeat with two more, or continue with the first a little longer.

Top Tip:

There are many combinations of any two exercises that can be applied, pick ones using the same muscles for growth or opposites for a fuller body workout but to reduce the rest time between sets try to think of two exercises that have a connecting point start and finish in the same place, eliminating the need to get up and re-position.

- Squat thrusts into tuck jumps
- Pushups into squat thrusts
- Sit ups into pike sit ups
- Plank into bear crawl

9. How to Get Incredible Results in Minutes! (Not hours)

Myth: Half an hour of running will always be better than 15 minutes for general fitness or fat burning

Truth: Not if you use the 15 minutes correctly!

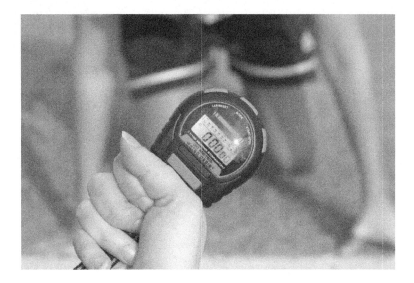

- "Use 'Interval' training to blast your fitness in minutes, not hours"

This book is all about getting you the best fitness results in the minimum time and this technique epitomizes this approach.

It's an old concept that if something is good for you then doing it for longer will be better for you, but in the spirit of economy, and of this book, why waste an hour when you could get the same results (or better) in half that?

Interval training, sometimes called (High Intensity Interval Training – HIIT) is a fairly recent fitness discovery blowing many traditional ideas out of the water. Where old styles of training would encourage fitness through endurance over long periods of time, Interval Training uses short bursts of higher intensity exercise to achieve great results much more quickly.

This approach is perfect for those looking to hack down the exercise time while still getting all the benefits normally reserved for those spending hours in the gym.

The concept of Interval Training is simple;

1. **One short burst of exercise at around 90% your maximum effort. (E.g. sprinting for a minute)**
2. **One short low intensity 'rest' period. (E.g. slow jogging for a minute)**
3. **Repeat the first step again**
4. **Repeat the second step again**

Repeat the entire process three to five times with recovery in between.

The whole action of high energy work followed by low intensity recovery increases fitness and burns far more calories for the same period of time that steady moderate intensity exercise like normal running.

(A study from McMaster University, Canada demonstrated that a total of 2.5 hours of sprint interval training yielded the same muscular development changes as 10.5 hours of 'normal' endurance training AND gave the same endurance improvements)

This system can also be applied to any other aerobic exercise such as running, rowing, swimming or cycling.

Here is a great full-body workout in just 4 mins that burns as many calories as a 40-60 min run. (For full details of the exercises see my other books; Fighting Fit, Bodyweight Handbook or of course check each one online)

1. 0-20 secs – Squat Thrusts
2. 20-30secs – Rest
3. 30-50secs – Mountain Climbers
4. 50secs-1min – Rest
5. 1min – 1.20 – High Knees
6. 1.20 – 1.30 Rest
7. 1.30-1.50 Jumping Jacks
8. 1.50 – 2mins – Rest
9. 2.00 – 2.20 – Squat Thrusts
10. 2.20 – 2.30 – Rest
11. 2.30 – 2.50 Mountain Climbers
12. 2.50 – 3mins – Rest
13. 3.00 – 3.20 - High Knees
14. 3.20 – 3.30 – Rest
15. 3.30 – 3.50 Jumping Jacks
16. 3.50 – 4mins - Rest and done!

As you get used to this process your muscles learn to more efficiently use fats for energy and you develop leaner body tone in up to a fifth of the time you normally would using traditional techniques.

In today's time-strapped world interval training could be your answer to fitness fast!

Top Tip: Get warm, not injured

Because interval training throws you straight into intense exercise warming up is an absolute must. Some light jogging or movement gets your body prepared and reduces chance of injury.

10.   Start Drinking

Put the beer down. It's water that we need here.

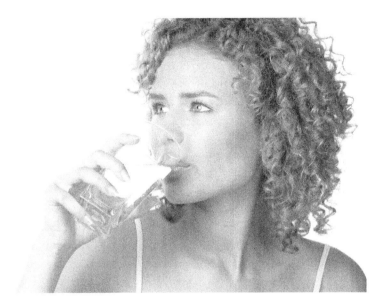

-   **"Consume the right amount of water and ignore the myths for optimal health"**

We all know that fluid replacement is important to maintain a healthy body but there are a lot of contrasting and pseudo-scientific claims about water consumption, suggesting everything from curing disease to damaging the heart.

While lots of people recommend 8 cups, or X amount of Litres a day the simplest way is to be governed by your thirst. Thirst starts to occur at around 2% below optimal hydration and so you have plenty of time to correct this.

On average the body uses 1 to 1.5 litres of water a day but the human body is very good at regulating water levels and we gain fluids from fruit, vegetables and even drinks like tea and coffee. Just necking litres of water each day is largely unnecessary unless you are in a hot climate or exerting yourself.

How to check:

The color of your urine is directly affected by how hydrated you are. If the pee is light and straw coloured you are probably ok. If it is dark yellow, like cider you are probably in need of some water.

Another of the most enduring rumours is that drinking a substantial amount of cold water first thing in the morning kick starts your metabolism and starts burning calories.

This is true, but only in the sense that you need water all the time anyway. Having a drink first thing helps restore fluid levels but only to the normal point that your body needs. As for burning calories the only way this would use more than the usual would be if the water was so cold that the body had to warm it up to body-temperature to use it. Yes a few more calories may be used but you would likely feel awful for a while so it's probably not worth it.

How much water do I need?

It is advised that at a minimum our body loses around 500ml of water a day through urine and around 700ml through breath and sweat.

With this in mind doctors suggest we should consume 1.2 Liters or 2.5 Pints of water (fluids) a day. Water is essential but there is no need to obsess over 8 glasses a day or some arbitrary figure. Your body will normally tell you when it's time to drink so try to pay attention to how you feel and use common sense.

Other Tips:

-   Skip the bottled water. Mineral water companies make millions every year selling their own unique take on thirst quenching but no evidence exists to support the benefits of bottled water over tap water. (Unless you live in places with unsafe mains water)
    In fact some studies suggest up to a quarter of bottled water is from a tap anyway!

-   On medication or eat a lot of salt? Increase your water intake to help your kidneys process the extra strain.

-   Drink to cure hunger. It sounds like a mix-up but some evidence shows the body has difficulty differentiating between an empty stomach through hunger and thirst. Many people swear that by having a glass of water when hunger hits and waiting 5 mins so you can see if it's just thirst making you feel that way.

Top Tip: Beat the heat with ice-cold water

Working out is usually hot, sweaty work, especially in warm countries. Beat the heat with ice water the right way. Put your water bottle in the freezer the night before you hit the gym or do your workout but only fill the bottle two-thirds full. Then, just before you leave to exercise, top the bottle up with normal water.

This not only gives you wonderfully refreshing water but it means you aren't struggling to get drinkable fluid from a solid block of ice!

Gym Hacks:

Sweaty individuals everywhere grunting with exhaustion and pain while perfect bodies all around make you feel bad about your own. No it's not that video I saw online once, it's the gym.

Love it or hate it the gymnasium is a big part of many people's lives and has in recent years become the staple of fitness in society, increasing year on year with over 50 Million health club members in the US alone according to the International Health, Racquet & Sports club Association.

Gyms are big business and like any product they have good and bad sides. Yes the equipment is all there and you have many options of classes, machines, weights and more. The price for all the fancy kit is of course the membership fees. Even a cheap pay-as-you-go type gym can cost hundreds every year. (I personally don't recommend these since it almost rewards you financially for NOT attending)

But the gym can be great too. Find a good one and you will be driven to work harder for longer and attend regularly, not to mention the benefits of working out with friends and the social interaction.

Hacking the gym is all about achieving the best results from your time there and getting the most bang-for-buck possible.

1. Get Through the Door

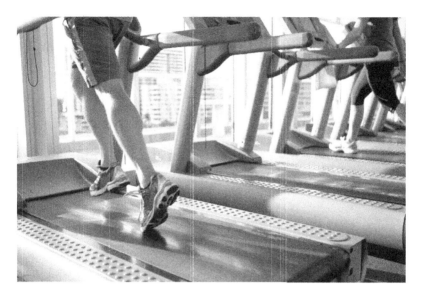

- *"Set foot through the door of your gym and half the battle is over!"*

The number one issue most people suffer with when it comes to Gym attendance is what is known as 'mental friction' or 'mental resistance'. The thought of attending the gym sits in your mind all day and meets more and more resistance until you eventually just skip it all together or find something that is definitely more important. (Re-arranging the sock drawer again eh?)

There are two ways to combat this and smooth out the friction. The first has already been discussed under *"Do it First"* chapter. This means that you basically do the things you don't want to do first thing in the day. Not only is early morning exercise more effective but you get the task out of the way and have the whole day stress free.

If you schedule gym at the end of the day there is the possibility of it being on your mind all day and building up resistance to the idea. Not only this but knowing you have to do something you aren't keen on will likely put you in a bad mood or distract you.

The second and personally my favorite approach is to simply agree to *'get through the door'*. This tactic could equally sit within **Mind Hacks** but the idea is simple; don't think about the workout you have to complete, don't think about the time you have to spend at the gym and don't even think about the exercises. Just focus on the simplest of tasks; getting through the door.

You can even tell yourself that you are just going to get through the door and see how you feel.

That's all.

No promises of exercise. No chiding yourself for not attending sooner. Just focus on one dead-easy task.

The beauty of course is that by nature once we walk through that door and see all the other folks sweating we feel foolish turning around to go home. It would be a wasted journey. At that point it makes far more sense to just crack on with it.

Even if you are dreading the workout, when you start you can promise yourself "just to do half today", again just focusing on a fraction of the normal amount. Once more we find that once the exercise is underway we feel far better and more motivated to finish it off fully.

So just 'get through the door' today.

Top Tip:

Feeling pushed for time? Not sure you'll get chance to work-out at the gym this morning but worried you might skip it altogether otherwise?

Swing by the gym first thing and leave your kit bag in your locker or behind the front desk, preferably with something important inside and tell them you will be back later for it.

When you return, after work for example, you've already overcome the hard part of getting through the door; you may as well do some exercise.

2. Upgrade to a Nicer Gym

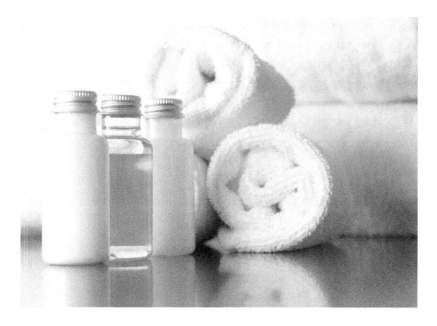

- *"Upgrade your gym experience and look forward to attending!"*

If you are lucky enough to have an overflowing bank account or at least a little extra in the budget to splurge on yourself, then consider a gym upgrade. Opt for an exclusive fitness center with all the bells and whistles. There is no way you will dread heading to the gym when stepping through those doors is just like entering a spa.

How would you like to feel as if you are on vacation, every time you work out?

While exclusive gym memberships can get a bit expensive, the motivational tradeoff is priceless. You will also notice that these types of centers provide unbeatable customer service. They want you to keep coming back, so they will do everything you can to make you feel welcome. This means you are less likely to feel intimidated by the overall experience.

Still worried about price? Let's take a look:

Say the average gym costs between 50 and 100 dollars a month (According to published figures)

That's 600 to 1200 dollars a year, which sounds like a lot but break it down to a daily cost and it works out at a maximum of around $3 per day.

Now consider your daily routine. Do you have a beer or glass of wine most nights while sitting around? Eat some donuts or junk food regularly? (50 Million Americans do on a daily basis) How much did you spend on these?

What about medicines? Do you take anti-depressants? Or diet pills?

What if instead of fuelling your unhealthy lifestyle and feeling worse about yourself every day you could go to a swanky establishment and use state of the art equipment to look better, feel better and meet new people?

Long term gym usage in most cases actually costs less than the alternative when you break it down and you are left fitter and happier in your daily life.

Although this one is not possible for everyone, if you can swing it, and it helps you stick to your fitness commitment, then go for it. Your health is one of the few things in which you will never regret investing.

Take advantage of all the extras, too. Most premium gyms include nice indoor pools, massages, free quality shampoos in the showers, and softer, more luxurious towels than any of the budget gyms provide.

But what if the cost of the gym is still just out of reach? There are still options…

3. Use Your Boss

Not like that, what kind of book do you think this is?

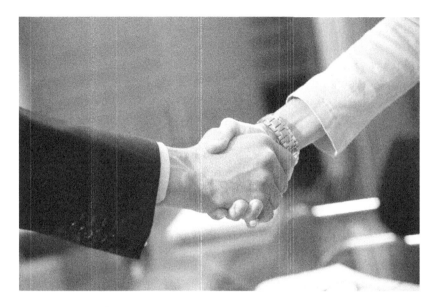

-*"Get discount gym membership through your employer"*

No, this tip is simply about making the most of your job.

If you work for a large company look into the company benefits. Most companies that employ many people offer some kind of fitness schemes. Be that their own on or off site gym or discounts for joining a local gym.

The best thing is that because companies are keen to appeal to new employees and prospective investors the gyms they associate with are usually high quality premium establishments.

A lot of companies also have discounts or free memberships for local sports associations or health clubs. Not interested in the gym? How about a discounted massage?

If your company doesn't have any system like this in place contact the HR department or 'Personnel' if they are old-school and make enquiries. You can even pitch the idea to them if no system is in place.

Companies typically care about the benefit to them, not to the employees. Cynical, perhaps, but also true. With this in mind structure your pitch around the long term benefits to employee satisfaction and productivity. A healthy, fit employee is one free of stress and with stress responsible for an estimated 40% of workplace absences you should be sure to point out the benefits to company and employee alike.

Just make sure to make your case with hard facts and figures to back up these claims. Print off a few example studies or capture some bookmarked websites showing the effects of exercise on office health before you suggest the idea to HR.

4. Hack Your Gym Fees Down

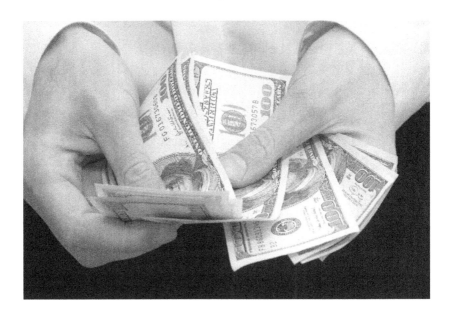

- *"Slash your gym fees, save money or get freebies by negotiating with the sales team"*

It's a funny thing about living in the West that we see a price on something and accept it, yet if you visit the Middle East or parts of Asia bartering over how much you pay is not only accepted it is almost expected!

The same is true of Gym memberships – though hardly anyone knows this. You, the client, or potential client have much more buying power than you may think.

Gyms are frantic to get you to sign up because a contract means recurring, guaranteed payments, just like a cell phone deal. And, just like a cell phone, there is a lot of room to negotiate on how much you pay per month.

Haggling is perfectly acceptable and even a small monthly discount can mean hundreds saved over the year for the sake of just one conversation. Go into it in a relaxed, happy manner. Getting aggressive or angry will just get you nowhere.

For existing members considering renewing:

- Always note in your diary when your membership is due to expire.

- Gather research about the other offers local gyms offer (or the offers for new members at your current gym)

- With a few weeks to go arrange to speak to one of their sales team, a supervisor or someone who can make the decisions – not a receptionist, and say you'd like to discuss renewing your membership.

- When you get to talk mention that you'd like to renew for another 12 months but you've seen some excellent local offers and ask if they can beat it.

- If they say no, remind them how much of a loyal customer you've been and that money is tight at the moment but you would be prepared to sign for a full year if they can do "x" off the price. (Work this out in advance)

- If they still won't budge ask about other benefits. Could you get a free upgrade, free passes for friends or free sports gear?

For prospective new members:

- Always try a one-day free trial to get a feel for a potential gym

- Compare other local gyms and try to find one or two with cheaper rates and note this down. Research is king.

- Call the nicest gym you are most interested in and ask if they have any offers on membership currently since you were recommended their establishment.

- If they say no, ask about other benefits of membership like free towels or sports gear etc.

- Ask if they can do any discount if you sign up today. If they agree then go ahead and feel free to sign up if you wish.

- If they show any wavering but uncertainty there is a good chance you will be able to sway them in person. Arange a time to go in, get a tour and speak one-to-one to someone who has the ability to make these decisions. (As mentioned before a supervisor or customer service rep is a good choice)

- As for existing members try to negotiate on the monthly rate, freebies or discounts on short term contracts depending on how often you plan to use the place.

- Offering to sign up there and then can give you bargaining power.

Remember:

- Some gyms are more open to negotiating than others but if you don't try you don't know.

- Go into the haggling with a smile and friendly approach. Look at it as a fun game

- Do your research and ideally have evidence to show of competitor prices

- Even saving just $10 a month saves you hundreds each year.

5. Use the Buddy System

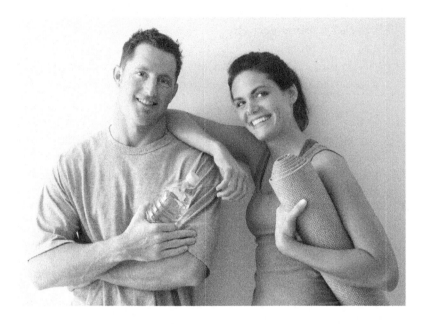

- *"Grab a friend and studies show you are more likely to stick to your commitments and work harder during exercise"*

Working on your own personal fitness goals does not mean you have to go it alone. Paring up with a friend is proven to increase your chance at success.

Studies indicate that through social accountability (telling people) we are more likely to stick to our promises, add the element of mild competition and having a friend present for exercise session becomes a powerful tool to increase fitness.

Choose a friend that you enjoy being around, and who has a similar level of commitment to exercising. Help each other stay motivated through the ups and downs of your fitness journey. Plus, your workouts will be much more fun when they double as social events.

Here are five more reasons to get a workout buddy:

1. You will not be as tempted to skip your workout session when someone else is counting on you to be there. This means you will work out more often, and stay committed for a longer period. You might even find yourself open to greater intensity levels than you expected.

2. Sometimes being accountable to yourself just is not enough. You can help each other stay on track with your diets as well by making healthy choices together. You will not feel like the odd man out choosing a salad when everyone else is binging on double cheeseburgers.

3. The time will race by when you are in good company. You can chat and share the latest gossip while you move through your sets. You will distract each other's attention away from the clock. You may even find yourself looking forward to your next workout session.

4. Your buddy is your second set of eyes. They may offer a more accurate assessment of your progress. They will notice when your strength and endurance begin to improve. You might even hear them compliment you after losing weight or gaining muscle. You can help each other stay positive by noticing the small achievements along the way. Boost each other's self-esteem.

5. Enjoy rewards together. Sit down and set some mini-goals worth achieving. Find healthy ways to celebrate as you pass each milestone. A few good options include not skipping any workouts for a month, losing ten pounds or a couple inches, or shaving a minute off your mile run. Treat yourselves to a movie, small shopping spree, spa night, or a drink at the bar as a reward. Just make sure the rewards you choose do not sabotage your progress.

6. How to Avoid the No.1 Weight Mistake

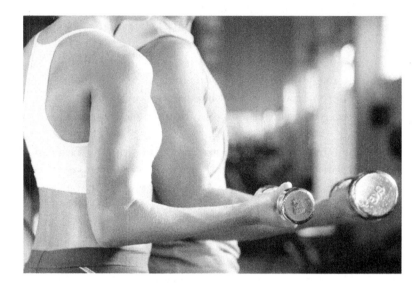

- *"Lift heavier weights for improved muscle tone, quicker. Ignore the myths surrounding weights"*

It's time to address one of the most popular myths in fitness. Lifting heavy weights DOES NOT lead to huge bulky muscles – if you don't want it to. This is a popular fallacy based on what seems to make sense to many people but in reality the results do not correlate.

Many women, for example, traditionally avoid heavy weights for fear of over-developed muscles and a beefed up appearance but that is extremely unlikely to occur unless you are dedicated to huge muscle growth as a goal.

Firstly it's worth understanding that due to the much lower testosterone levels, (on average around 15 times lower) found in women, the muscle growth following weight sessions will not be as pronounced as men. This makes it much harder for women to get 'big' but easier to get 'toned'.

In fact lifting heavy is beneficial for men and women as an efficient way to become leaner and stronger in a quicker space of time.

Lifting lighter weights can increase muscular endurance but lifting heavy tones the body in the way most people want by increasing muscle density creating a tighter appearance. (It's worth also noting that fat cannot be converted into muscle. You can lose fat and build muscle, both will help but one does not become the other.)

Your body also burns more calories maintaining muscle than it does for fat and so the more muscle fibers you have the higher your metabolism and the better you look. (If weight loss is your game).

It's also the reason that as you get fitter you may need to consume more calories. Don't assume this is a bad thing; your body needs them to fuel your new leaner body. (But of course calories from healthy food works better).

So should I ditch lighter weights altogether?

It's up to you depending on how long you wish to spend down the gym. In studies carried out by McMaster University they found the point in which muscle tone starts to increase is only found when you workout a muscle to the point of fatigue – when you literally cannot lift another repetition. To reach this point with heavier weights is quicker and easier but you could do it with light weights if you have a lot of time.

In summary;

- 'Toning' as a term generally means, lower body fat and increased muscle density

- Lifting heavier weights is recommended for both men and women

- Heavier weights do not cause major 'bulking up' unless that is your goal and it requires major diet and exercise changes to do this.

- Lifting heavier weights for fewer repetitions produces increased muscle tone quicker than an extended light-weight workout.

- Lifting heavy increases strength, whereas light increases endurance

- Lift until point of fatigue (when you cannot lift more) to improve muscle growth

So next time you hit the gym don't be afraid of the heavy weights.

7. New Clothes: New Motivation

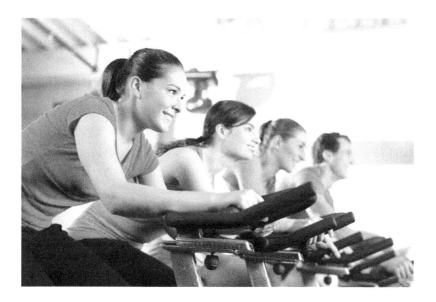

- "Pick up some new workout clothes for instant exercise motivation!"

Purchasing new workout clothing may seem shallow but it is about more than just looking good. Have you ever purchased a new car and felt like you can't wait to drive it? Or bought a new suit or dress and instantly felt smarter or more attractive? The same is true for gym-wear and the way we present ourselves directly affects how we feel.

New clothes feel good and they will also help you be more confident and ready to tackle your next fitness challenge. Not only this but dressing the part is an instant boost to feeling the part.

While the fancier outfits might catch your eye, you really do not need to spend a lot to get a few new workout outfits. The trick is to look for fabrics that breathe and fit you well to boost confidence. Once you find some new clothes that you love, you will be excited to wear them for your next workout. In addition to this motivational factor, choosing workout clothes is downright fun.

If you dress sporty, you will feel sporty. Even if you aren't a natural athlete you can 'fake it until you make it' by using the age-old principal of acting the part until you eventually become the part.

If you are a runner, or just tend to sweat, a lot while exercising then you might want to look into clothing with a bit of technology. Today there are a variety of fabrics like Coolmax, designed to whisk sweat away from your skin for a more comfortable experience. You will feel more confident too. Besides, once you put on those clothes you really cannot just lounge around the house, you will instantly feel the urge to get active.

Schedule a new shopping trip every 6 months and if you are looking to lose weight or perhaps gain muscle consider buying the size you aspire to and working towards fitting in that outfit. Of course always get fit for your own reasons and being healthy is far more important than fitting in some outfit.

Top Tip:

Leave your workout clothes either next to your bed, next to your alarm or somewhere you cannot miss them. The first instinct when waking up will be to put them on.

8. Get Paid for Working Out!

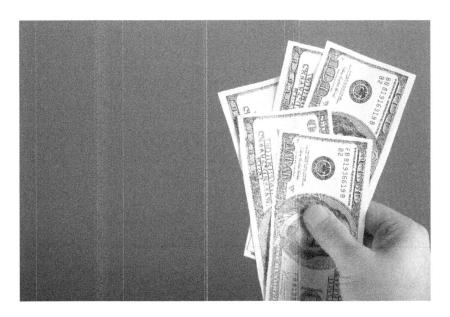

- *"Use a 'fund' or special App and get paid for attending the gym!"*

Money is a big motivator in life.

You may not like your job very much or perhaps you truly enjoy it. Either way, you probably would list it fairly high on your priority list. When the alarm starts to beep and you do not want to get out of bed, you reluctantly wake up anyway.

While pride or personal satisfaction may play a part in this decision, one of your biggest motivators is probably the check you receive at the end of each pay period. Even when you just do not feel like going in, you still do because working will help you acquire the things you want or need in life.

Why not apply this same strategy to working out? Would you be more likely to stand by your fitness commitment if you got paid every time you worked out? What if you got paid extra for overtime? If this sounds good to you, then find a jar, a small box, or even a plain white envelope and begin paying yourself. For each completed workout, add one or two dollars to your fund. You can include an additional bonus when you go the extra mile.

Let the money accumulate for four to six months. Then use it to splurge on something extra special. You can spend your money on whatever you like, but some great ideas include new workout clothes, a pair of sneakers, a new water bottle, or music. Watching the bills add up will motivate you to keep going. You will be less likely to skip your workouts, and more likely to put in a few extra reps as you daydream about your reward.

While shedding pounds, sculpting, and building strong muscles is a reward in itself, it is always nice to have a little extra incentive. Reward yourself for all of your hard work!

Ok, so giving yourself some money after a workout is cool but what if someone else was giving it to you?

Even better right?

The easiest way to do this is to set up an agreement with a close friend - preferably someone you regularly workout with anyway since they can monitor your progress. (And check you aren't being dishonest!).

Give your friend a small but significant amount of money each month and ask them to hold on to this. Each time you complete a gym session ask them to give you some of the money back. Or, at the end of the month agree that you get money back based on how often you attended the gym.

This money can be part of a 'fun fund' that you can spend on things you enjoy. The beauty of this tactic is that it reinforces the positive sensation of attending the gym and subconsciously associates it with a good feeling (getting paid).

If you want to go hardcore and really push your motivation allow your friend to keep any of the money that isn't returned to you at month's end. Suddenly you will find your gym attendance improves drastically!

Apps

Many Apps exist to help you with the Gym but a few have taken a clever financial approach to improving motivation.

Apps like 'GymPact' use a similar approach to the 'Fun Fund' previously mentioned. GymPact takes your credit card details when you sign up and tracks your attendance based on signing in to gym locations through Wifi or GPS. Should you miss the gym session you agreed to your card is charged $5 minimum for the indiscretion.

But good news! If you do attend the gym as agreed you actually *receive* money into your account; a portion of the very same funds taken from others around the world who haven't attended that day.

If you are wondering if it's possible to make a profit from this approach well yes, in theory, but the amounts involved are quite small and the hours required in the gym would be massive to produce anything worthwhile!

That said the principal of financial motivation is always a powerful one so try it out for your gym attendance today.

9. Listen To a Story

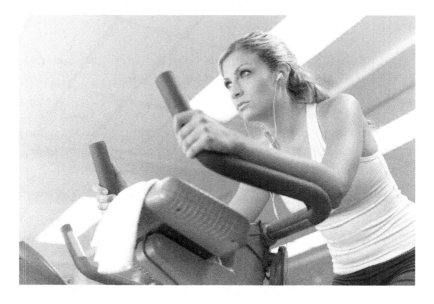

- *"Listen to an Audiobook or Podcast while you Exercise and get hooked on working out!"*

Combine two great pastimes for one mega workout boost!

Seek a fascinating audio book or podcast that you may enjoy. Look for podcasts related to your interests, or specifically designed to help you through your fitness hurdles. Alternatively, find an audio book that corresponds with a novel you have been meaning to read.

Now, declare that you will not by any means listen to your newfound pleasure unless you are being physically active. This will provide a helpful little shove towards your workout. You may even find yourself performing an extra set or two so that you can complete the current chapter or discussion.

There are dozens of podcasts designed for just this reason. They will keep you engaged and motivated without distracting from the task at hand. Challenging exercises will bring less discomfort and the time will fly right by as you listen.

These types of mediums are great if you are looking for a workout partner that is more stimulating than music, but not as distracting as television. By listening to a podcast or audio book, you will stimulate your mind, making double use of your time.

Take your chosen book or podcast for a test run. While any selection will do the trick, some are certainly better than others. Make sure the speaker has pleasant, different, or distinct voice that will maintain your attention. Some listeners swear by unusual or sensual accents. Unfortunately, some selections can be downright boring or painful to hear for any duration. A quick test spin will ensure that your choice is a positive addition to your workout routine.

10. Look at Yourself

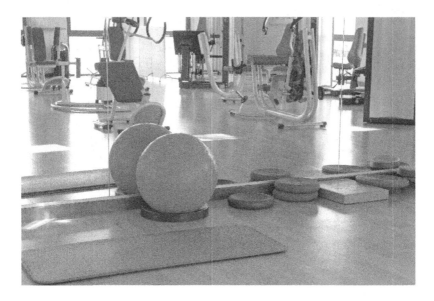

- *"Look in the mirror while you work out to improve form and reduce tiredness!"*

Most gyms include at least some sections of the wall covered in mirrors. Quite often this is around the free weights area but sometimes surrounding the treadmills and cross-trainers too.

Many people will rightly claim this is to improve assessment of form during technical lifts and exercises. Which is true - after-all once you are attempting to bench your own bodyweight one minor slip and you can do permanent damage.

The more cynical may argue that mirrors are also there for posers to look at themselves while they workout – possibly true also. But funnily enough this actually works, especially in the case of cardio.

Recent studies show that observing yourself performing an activity makes you work harder, have better form and feel less exhausted.

Research published in the Medicine & Science in Sports & Exercise Journal showed that runners were more relaxed, more motivated and ran with better form than runners who didn't have a mirror in front. Even better, it documented that they felt less tired after the exercise.

The theory is that the mirror not only allows a person to correct their form but doing this distracts them from the exhaustion and they feel much less fatigue.

Although the study sampled a fairly small group of individuals it is expected that the results would apply to anyone, especially runners, involved in any exercise that can improve with correct form.

So next time you hit the treadmill or weights bench don't be afraid to take a look in the mirror. It's not just for posers!

Hacks At Home:

A lot of people don't feel comfortable working out with others and they can't afford a fancy gym so what options are there for keeping in shape at home?

Of course you can create a home-gym room, clear the space for weights or buy a home cross-trainer but far better is to introduce simple, effective changes that don't require the complete overhaul of your abode.

Your house might not seem like the center of wellbeing, with the TV, Computers and Sofa, but with a few small tweaks you can develop habits that use your daily routine for your fitness benefit.

Either as stand-alone tips or as a boost to your gym/exercise sessions the following tricks are designed to be easily integrated with the things you do every day.

1. Skip the Gym (Wait, what?)

Here's the honest truth; you do not need to go to the gym to get fit.

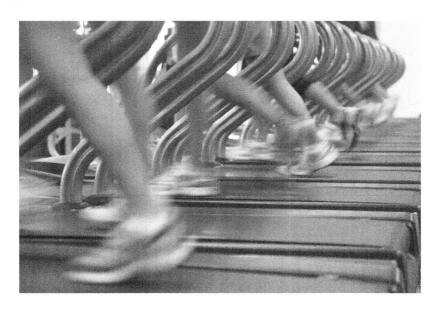

- *"Skip the gym and you may exercise more!"*

You may be surprised that I am starting this section by suggesting people skip the gym but the fact remains that through extensive marketing and many preconceptions the fitness companies and gyms do an excellent job of making the general public believe that their way is the only way. It works for many, but may not be for you.

Getting hung up on working out in a gym setting can even sabotage your goals in some cases. If you live a busy life like many of us, there may not be enough hours in the day to make it to the gym regularly. This means you might find yourself skipping your workout all together. Yet if you take the gym out of the equation, it will become easier to sneak a twenty-minute workout into even the busiest of days.

1. While the gym may seem convenient for some people, you might feel intimidated as a beginner. It is also normal to be confused about how all the complicated looking equipment works. If you do feel uncomfortable at the gym, you will be more likely to skip it all together. The best way to guarantee that your fitness journey is a success is by choosing a process that you truly enjoy.

If you are shy, or feel self-conscious around all those perfect bodies, you might have trouble focusing on your own workout at the gym. If stepping in to the gym makes you nervous, skip it and choose to workout in the comfort of your own home.

2. While the personal trainer at your gym might be full of information, they can sure be pricey. You can get equal results in your home or at the park. Purchase a workout DVD if you prefer step-by-step guidance without the hefty price tag.

3. You really do not need any of those large and complicated machines. Keep it simple with sets of pushups, or crunches. If you have a few dollars to spend, invest in free weights, resistance bands, or an exercise mat. If money is tight, you can skip this expense by using bodyweight exercises (http://bit.ly/1ncr5y2), or by lifting household items such as canned goods or laundry detergent instead.

4. You might be happier if you can get outside. Fresh air is a great way to fuel your workout. Take a walk or jog around the neighborhood. The cheaper and simpler your workout is the more likely you will be to stick with it.

5. If you do not like the gym, or have trouble finding the motivation to get there, and then give yourself permission to skip it. There are other ways to get where you are going. You might find it is easier to find the motivation to simply stand up from the couch and get going, than to make the arduous trip across town to the fitness studio.

6. At home you can listen to your favorite music, as loud as you choose. Or, you can watch your favorite show while you complete your reps. It also does not matter what you wear in the privacy of your house.

7. Even if the gym does work for you, you might find it fun to perform a home workout occasionally. Variety can really help you stick with your fitness commitment.

2. Play Video Games to Get Fit

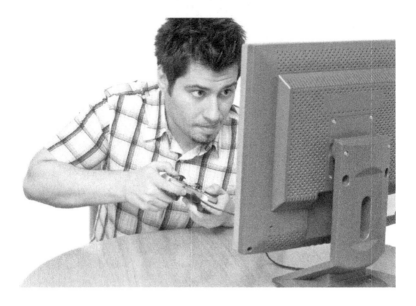

"Use the power of motion in video games to get in shape, or just stand up!"

A lot of people love video games and I'm not ashamed to say on occasion I'm one of them. The combination of action, adventure, problem solving and great story telling is purposely built to be addictive. Little wonder then that the video games industry is valued at more than the film and music industry combined! Incredible stuff.

Unfortunately sitting on your backside bashing a controller has never helped you get in shape and traditionally the better you are in the virtual world the worse your fitness in the real world.

At least until recently.

It was only a few years ago we marveled at the special effects of movies like Minority Report which depicted people controlling futuristic looking computers by moving their arms around and directing the screen.

Fast forward a few years; the technology has caught up and this is now reality. (Does this mean we can soon expect personalized jet-packs?!) In any case, with Microsoft, Nintendo and Sony developing the 'Kinect', 'Wii' and 'Move' technology we suddenly have a way to actively participate in video games using our whole body.

This is perfect for you video game fans who can now engage your muscles while fighting the dark side, fending off marauding Orcs or running explosive military operations in far flung locations.

But it's not just for the traditional 'geeks'. A quick look at the motion-based games available on the various platforms reveal every kind of genre you could imagine. So even if the idea of running around shooting and blowing stuff up doesn't interest you there is the chance to play puzzle games, racing games, historical simulations or even pure fitness challenges.

Yes, there is also a dedicated genre for those who just wish to get fit. These 'games' will engage your body in everything from Cardio and weightlifting to Yoga and Dance, all monitored by your console and all available in the comfort of your own home!

Perfect for people of all ages and fitness levels video games are the new fitness revolution.

But what if I don't have one of those consoles?

Even if you don't have a motion based games system there is a easy way to improve your fitness while playing; just stand up.

While you bash the controller and vanquish your enemies make sure you are standing as you face the screen, not slumped on a sofa. The simple act of standing up is shown to have great health benefits and as we will discover later burns thousands of calories more over a year.

Top Tip: Loading screen lunges

If you play a game with detailed graphics, lots of different levels and characters chances are there will be a 'loading' screen or similar while your computer or console loads the next area. Use this time to perform 'loading lunges'.

Complete a lunge on one leg, then alternate to the next and repeat one on each side for as long as it takes to load. These are great since you can perform them upright and while watching the screen so you don't miss a second of the action.

3. Watch Television

Ok, so video games make some sense but you're probably wondering how watching TV can possibly help you get fit.

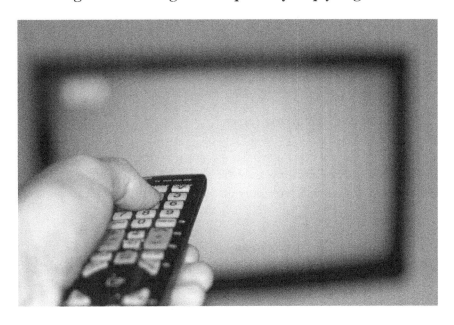

- *"Introduce 'games' to your TV habit and get fit while watching."*

While watching television may not be perceived as the healthiest habit, it might be one worth trying with a twist. This does not mean you should become a couch potato. Instead, focus on a favorite film, series or both. If you do not have one, then explore the options until you find something to your liking.

The process is about setting rules and making it a game for yourself, a little like the way drinking games sometimes work. Not that any of us would know about such things of course...

Essentially you get your favorite TV show on the go then decide on a certain cue to engage in exercise. The cue could be anything but think about how often and how long you wish to workout.

Example one: The catchphrase game

In this example you agree to perform say, 10 pushups, every time a character says or does something they are known to do.

Let's say you decide to do 10 pushups each time Homer does something stupid in The Simpsons.

Example two: Ad break exercises

If you watch a show on normal TV promise yourself to jog on the spot during each time the commercials are shown. Even at 2 minutes per set and 3 repetitions each 30 minutes you are completing 6 minutes of jogging.

Example Three: Serial Exercise

Watch a show you love and know you will get hooked on.

Next, set a rule that you cannot watch the next episode unless you are active for a set duration – say 10 minutes.

You can burn a good amount of calories during that time. Choose one or more simple activities, which you can easily accomplish without too much thought.

Avoid movements that require precise positioning. Instead, look for a fun option such as skipping rope, jumping on a small workout trampoline, dancing around, performing the running man, or play with a hula-hoop. It should be fun after all!

If strength training is more your game, try some basic free-weight exercises. Try to swap in something a bit more challenging during the commercials. By tying in your favorite sitcoms, your workout will become associated with something more pleasant. The time will also fly by, and you will not be staring at the clock during your routine. More importantly, you will not be as tempted to skip your session if it means you also have to miss the show.

4. Share Online

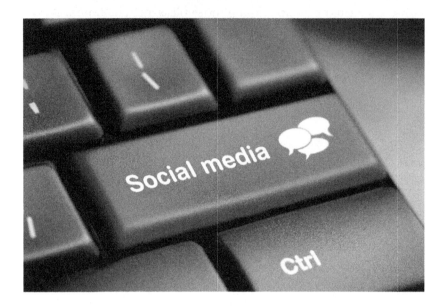

- *Tell people and use 'Social Accountability' for powerful motivation"*

Have you ever agreed to get up early or do something difficult for a friend, family member or co-worker? Did you notice how you accepted this and got on with it?

This comes down to 'social accountability' or put another way; we feel much more inclined to do something if we have told others we would. Use this principal online for exercise inspiration.

By sharing your fitness goals and progress online, you will find yourself more motivated than ever. You can be as open or anonymous as you wish. In fact, you might feel more comfortable sharing under a secret screen name than chatting your real life friends, and that is okay. Develop an online support network to share in your successes and catch you when you fall.

One way to do this is by joining a fitness forum. There are countless choices available so do some research and choose the best fit for your personality. Avoid boards and forums that seem bombarded with drama. Seek out a supportive environment instead. As you become more familiar with your new group, you may enjoy posting your personal results at the end of each week. With this practice, you will become more accountable to yourself as well as to your new friends.

If you would like more control in your online sharing venue, and have an interesting story to tell, consider beginning a blog. You can do this instead of or in addition to joining a forum; it is all up to you. With a blog, you can introduce yourself to your readers. It can be shared with all of your family members and friends, or stay undercover with a new alias if that makes you feel more comfortable. Post your progress, short and long-term goals, admit to your mistakes, and highlight your achievements.

A regularly updated blog will attract readers who can share in your journey, offer advice, and find motivation to jumpstart their own fitness improvements. Every few months, look back to your earlier posts for a clear view of how far you have come. This will become a great resource as you review your past goals and evaluate how to progress towards a fitter future.

Finally you can also tag your locations and progress throughout Twitter, Facebook and other social networks. By announcing your intentions and progress to the world there is an increased audience pushing you to succeed.

5. How One Change to Your Workspace Can Burn Thousands of Calories!

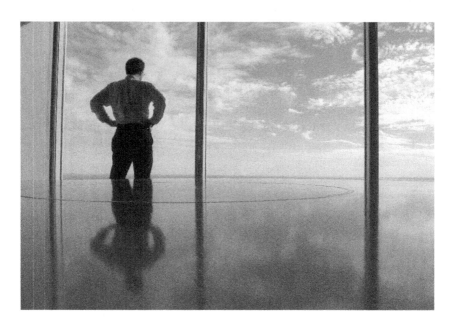

- *"Stand up more or tweak your workspace for drastic fitness improvements!"*

Maybe you work at home, maybe you don't, but chances are you spend a large portion of each week in your employment and probably staring at a digital screen in some form or another. An estimated two thirds of all Americans use a computer on a daily basis for work, but a bad workspace is literally killing you slowly.

Luckily one simple trick has been shown to change all that.

Stand up for fitness.

Just the act of standing up for a small portion of your day has been proven to make a massive difference to the long term health of employees.

A BBC study conducted in conjunction with the University of Chester showed that office workers standing instead of sitting for just 3 hours a day would, over the course of a year, have lowered the chance of heart disease and burned around 30,000 calories or 8lbs of fat.

(That's about the equivalent of running 10 Marathons!)

This evidence indicates that you don't even need to switch to all-day standing. By switching just 40% of your office time to standing up the health improvements are measureable with increased calorie burn and better bodily processing of blood sugar.

Try to spend more time on your feet and see the benefits.

But I can't stand up in my job…

Standing desks or standing workspaces are great but sometimes just not possible. If this is the case you can still smarten up your working experience and improve your health with these quick tricks;

Posture
The position you adopt while on a computer, or any job, is incredibly important. Take a look now and consider how you sit at work.

Feet
Your feet should be flat on the floor and your seat adjusted so you don't need to lean or shuffle forward to achieve this.

Shoulders
Shoulders should be relaxed, not up by your ears. Drop the arms of your chair so your shoulders can relax fully.

Sit up straight-ish

Research has shown that actually sitting bolt upright isn't the best position for your body while using a computer. In fact the ideal form is roughly 135 degrees according to numerous studies but this can be unrealistic for many people. Instead try to keep your body upright, but not rigid.

Avoid the hunch

One of the worst, yet sadly most common, positions seen in an office environment is the hunched over the keyboard position. From the side the spine may resemble a question mark. If you feel this forming take a second to straighten up.

20-20-20

For every 20 minutes of staring at a screen take 20 seconds off to look at something 20 feet away. This gives the eyes a break and chance to focus on something else reducing eyestrain.

Don't skip lunch

The British Chiropractic Association reported that roughly 50% of people don't leave their desk even for lunch, but this rest period and the break from screen time is important for a healthy back and eyes. Consider which is more important to you; getting that little extra work done now or years of pain and difficulty later in life.

Stand when you can

So you can't stand up at your desk. What about standing or walking during lunch? Or whilst watching a presentation or talking to someone? Even little changes from sitting to standing make long term improvements to health.

Gym Balls

For a long time many fitness experts and doctors have recommended a gym-ball (sometimes called a Swiss Ball or Yoga Ball) instead of a regular chair for computer use. The logic is sound; sitting on a slightly unstable platform like a ball forces your body to make hundreds of tiny, almost unperceivable adjustments to stay upright – hence working your core muscles all day and improving your posture.

The trouble is that the evidence is mixed regarding the efficacy of this technique. Yes, many people swear by it and the improvements to their body, yet others claim it made things worse and ultimately revert back to regular chair use.

Even the scientific results are unclear in this case with studies showing both positive and negative outcomes for each investigation. Ultimately the gym-ball <u>may</u> work for you but it's recommended you gradually introduce the new seating arrangement before you throw out the old chair.

- Again keep your feet flat on the floor for stability
- Ensure you have the right sized ball for you
- Keep in inflated
- Try for an hour at a time to begin, gradually increasing duration

Exercise balls are not for everyone and for each account of one fixing someone's posture and improving their core strength there are others of people finding them annoying and difficult to use with little to no benefit.

Try it out for yourself but do give it a fair go. Test for perhaps two weeks and at the end take stock of your natural seated posture and comfort level. If you find it hasn't really helped at work you can always switch back to a normal chair and take the ball home for use while exercising or watching TV.

6. Supercharge Your Walk

Walking seems like it wouldn't do much at all. Most of us do it every day and don't give it a second thought but of course like any physical activity it burns calories.

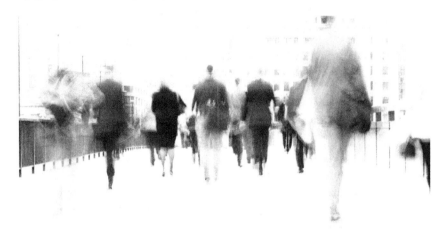

- *"Alter your walk and boost the workout"*

Because we generally don't associate walking with exercise it can be an effective way to trick our minds into getting active without the associated inner groan of resistance. So just how many calories can I burn walking?

As you'd expect it's not as many as running but it's still not bad.

The following figures are based on an **average male**, around **37/38 years old**, around **170llbs,** completing the exercises for an hour.

Calories listed are Calories burned per hour.

(Remember these are ROUGH guidelines and results are totally individual. If you are heavier or find the exercises harder you will use more calories and vice versa for lighter/fitter individuals)

Running / Jogging		Calories Burned Per Hour
Running at approx.	5 mph	644
Running at	7 mph	959
Running at	10 mph	1,260
Running a	5.5 minute mile	1,301
Walking		
Walking	2 to 3 mph	189
Walking	5 mph	531

So what if there was a way to improve the effects of walking without breaking into a run? Good news, there is.

Don't use your arms.

Or more accurately, **don't swing them.**

Swinging your arms aids the body in the natural gait during walking. As revealed in a recent study, arm motion is actually an evolutionary development improving our movement, not a left-over remnant from our primate ancestors.

The study outlined in *Proceedings of the Royal Society B (Biological Sciences)* at The University of Michigan investigated the effects of arm swinging via evolutionary biology and through measuring human walking with no swinging, over swinging and opposite arm swinging.

While many conclusions were drawn the most interesting may be that by keeping the arms steady at your side you increase the effort of walking by approximately 12%. This translates to the same energy as walking 20% faster or carrying a 10kg weight around.

The arms don't need to be over-tense, just held loosely at the body's side without swinging.

The study also showed that swinging the arms out-of-synch with the legs created an even greater effort and calorie burn however this, from a practical standpoint, makes for a difficult exercise to maintain. Not to mention the fact you may look like a crazy person!

So the next time you take a stroll in the park, to the shops or even just around the house try it without moving your arms and get a better workout.

Top Tip:

If you have a little cash to spend you can also buy ankle or wrist weights. These comfy bands typically add a small amount of weight to your limbs and you go about normal activity unaware you are working that little bit harder than normal.

7. Brush Your Teeth and Build Muscle

If you are doing it properly you probably spend a couple of minutes in the morning and a couple in the evening brushing your teeth. Why not use that time?

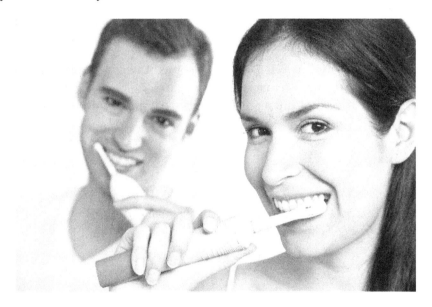

-"Use your toothbrush time to quietly build muscle by balancing"

This quick little hack is extremely simple.

While you stand there brushing raise the knee and lift one leg off the ground and hold for approximately one minute. If you wish, try tucking it against the standing knee in a Yoga-esque pose. After a minute swap legs and repeat on the other side.

Just the simple act of balancing engages many of your core muscles and activates many areas not used in normal daily life.

If you are using a non-electric toothbrush this creates even more of an exercise as you balance against the movement of the brush.

This type of toothbrush yoga is best applied as part of a regular habit but should be easy since there is normally nothing else to do during this time.

You can also make it a touch more intense by slightly lowering and raising the body while on the one leg, performing a very shallow squat motion.

You aren't going to get ripped using this approach and you won't exactly lose weight but you can engage some often-overlooked muscles and if you adopt it as a habit, which is key to long term success, it can be effective as part of the many little tricks for improving your body listed elsewhere.

Important:

If you are even slightly unsure of your balance don't try this one without being extra careful.. Working muscles is great but slipping over and/or swallowing your toothbrush is not. Take care with this exercise.

Top Tip:

Another approach is to brush normally but instead of rinsing with water simply spit out the excess and let the remaining toothpaste do its job afterwards while you maintain the single leg pose for a minute or two.

Many experts suggest that rinsing with water after brushing removes all the protective fluoride and that keeping it there, even for a short period, is better for your mouth.

8. The No.1 Tactic for Beating Stress

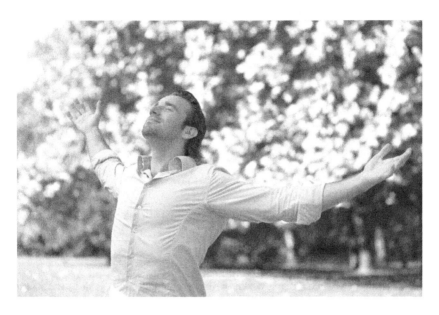

- *"Learn 'proper breathing' to banish stress and aid fitness"*

If Fitness is the goal then stress is the enemy.

Stress is probably the single biggest enemy of fitness. Stress is linked to a huge percentage of illnesses and if we consider being 'fit' as being in the best possible shape to complete the things you need to do on a daily basis then stress is the biggest obstacle to that.

The Health and Safety Executive in the UK reports around 40% of all work-related illness is stress related while in the U.S the American Psychological Association, American Institute of Stress, NY detail that an incredible 77% of individuals "regularly experience physical symptoms caused by stress".

With these worrying figures it's important to have simple tools at your fingertips to manage stress whenever it arises.

There are many different ways of managing stress and you can of course test various techniques to find the one that resonates most with you but the in the spirit of cutting through the superfluous and getting straight to the tips that work, the simplest method proven to consistently work is the one you should turn to first. And that is to breathe.

It sounds stupid discussing how to breathe, we're all doing it now after all but incredibly most people do it wrong. Or at least it could be better.

Take the test right now:

- Take a deep breath and notice how your body moves.
- Did your chest inflate?
- Did your shoulders rise?

In fact the motion of your upper body has very little to do with taking a deep breath, it's just that we associate the motion with breathing.

The diaphragm is the muscle responsible for drawing air into the lungs and it is situated much lower than people think. It sits below the rib cage and just around the stomach region. To truly draw proper breaths it's important to focus on this area and try to visualize each breath in expanding the stomach area and each breath out shrinking it.

When Stress Hits:

- Try to become still physically (if possible)
- Draw your attention to your breath
- Focus on the air passing your lips and down into your lungs
- Focus on the air reaching lower into your stomach region
- Imagine a ball within your stomach, upon each inhalation try to inflate the ball. With each breath out it deflates.
- In between each breath hold for a couple of seconds

9. Trick Your Brain Into Eating Less With...

...Plates.

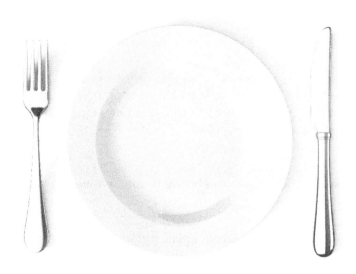

-    *"Adjust your dinnerware to feel fuller or reduce appetite!"*

Here's an unusual one but a trick that bizarrely works!

If you struggle at meal time to control how much you eat research suggests the type of dinnerware you use could make a big difference.

Specifically we are talking plates.

There are two tricks recently discovered to push your mind in the right direction when it comes to eating less, if you need to. The first is all about color.

Ever noticed how all the fast food companies seem to use the same color schemes in their logos? The reds and yellows of McDonalds, KFC and hundreds of others aren't coincidence. These are actually colors proven to increases heart rate, excitement and stimulate the appetite centers of the brain!

In fact a University of Toronto study showed that simply looking at Fast Food logos makes people more impatient and likely to go for a quick fix, than a slower healthier solution.

Conversely blue, as a color has been shown to reduce the craving for food.

With this in mind a dead-simple trick is to swap out your plain white or, god forbid, yellow plates and dishes for blue ones. While you may not consciously notice the difference studies have shown you should experience a reduction in appetite.

The second sneaky tip is to simply reduce your plate size to feel fuller.

It's obvious that having a smaller plate reduces your ability to pile up the food, there is less room, but it also has a psychological effect of still appearing to be a full plate of food to your brain.

Once you finish eating you will still feel full following the clean plate, even though the plate was smaller to start with.

10.   How to Clean Up Your Act

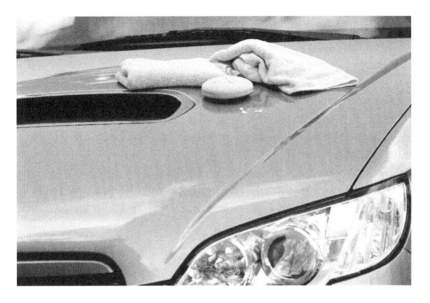

- *"Clean up your home, garden or car to burn calories!"*

A lot of people hate household chores but we realize that they need to be done anyway, hence we just get on with it. But most people don't realize that cleaning up around the home and garden is actually a great, low impact workout that burns calories.

Dusting, sweeping and mopping is an excellent way of generating a mild workout and if you increase the pace you can burn 4-6 calories a minute. Vacuuming, which typically utilizes a heavy vacuum device is also great for building arm strength as you move it around the house and burns even more.

Let's take an average person dusting as the simplest example:

- **4 Calories burned per minute**
- **20 minutes average, means 80 calories**

- At approximately one hour a week this burns 12,460 calories a year!
- Equivalent calorie burn as 4-6 Marathons run over 12 months!

But dusting is pretty easy, what if you'd like to take it further?

If you enjoy your car you can save money, have a sparkling ride and get in shape at the same time. Washing your car is slightly more intense than dusting around the house and is estimated to burn 6-8 calories per minute depending on speed.

Based on a 30 minute wash per week this results in approximately 9,360 calories burned over the year…and a whole lot of money saved by doing it yourself!

Top Tip:

If you want to make it a real workout simply increase the speed at which you work. Washing the car faster or cleaning around the house at an increased speed ups the calorie burn and increases endurance. For added motivation consider adding music.

Bonus! Don't forget that aside from getting a good workout you are also getting a clean and tidy home, garden or car, which in turn can improve your mood!

Cheating While Eating (Diet Hacks):

There is an old saying that "You can't work off a bad diet" and this is true. The fuel you put into your body powers your exercise after all, so putting the wrong stuff in instantly limits your physical ability from the outset.

A 2012 study carried out with the Hanza tribe of Tanzania, tracking their movement and energy usage showed that despite their traditional hunter-gatherer lifestyle and far more active existence as compared to the average office worker in the West, they did not exhibit a significantly higher metabolism as expected.

What does this mean? Essentially it shows that just being active and exercising more will not, alone, make you thin. Diet is just as important, if not more so.

The following tips focus on easy changes you can make to your daily eating habits without sacrificing the food you like to eat. Why? Because if you scrap **all** the food you enjoy there is an excellent chance you will fall of the wagon completely and disregard any healthy eating at all. As always small, manageable changes are important for long term success.

1. Go Bananas!

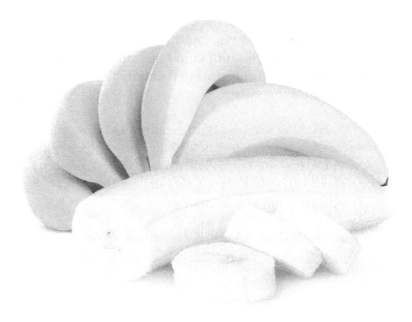

- *"Introduce a Banana a day to your diet for quick and easy health benefits"*

Diets are usually long winded complicated affairs involving lots of theory and understanding calories – which is why it's estimated 90% of people don't stick to them.

So what if I could give you one simple, cheap and effective tip to improve your diet right now? Well it would be mean not to after that build up so here it is:

Eat a Banana a day.

It's that simple. Eating one Banana a day can have significant impacts on improving your physical and mental health.

Yes, there are foods higher in antioxidants, certain vitamins, minerals and fiber and yes there are more popular 'superfoods', (but we'll get to those later) however for all-round health benefits and outright ease of use Bananas are hard to beat.

Remember the principle of this book is simple, effective and quick tips. If I told you that a rare Amazonian berry would fix your diet overnight it would do little good to 99% of the readers who live near supermarkets and towns.

Bananas on the other hand are easy to find, cheap, tasty, packed with nutritional benefits and proven to improve your mental health.

Yep, it's been proven that the little yellow guys are not just tasty and energy giving but proven to be effective at lifting mood. The British NHS even recommends Bananas as part of a healthier diet to combat symptoms of anxiety and depression.

Not only that but the World Health Organization found that people with a higher Potassium intake – a good source of which is bananas – had a 24% reduced risk of stroke. Of course like all things too much Potassium is bad for you but a single Banana a day can make a positive difference.

So go Bananas and feel better today!

2. Cheating Your Way To 5-A-Day

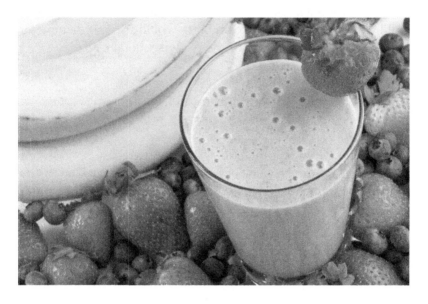

-   *"Get your recommended Fruit and Veg intake the easy way; through a daily smoothie"*

Although it goes under different names the '5-a-day' programme, sometimes called 'Fruits and Veg' or 'More matters' is a scheme that was set up in the UK, USA, Canada and a number of European countries to encourage increased consumption of Fruit and Vegetables within the general public.

Concerns arose several years ago when studies revealed the average Western household consumed far less than the recommended intake of vitamins and minerals, such as typically found in Fruit and Veg. The World Health Organization recommended that individuals take on at least 400g of vegetables daily and so governments responded by introducing these campaigns to push awareness for healthier living.

On paper this is a great idea. We already know that fruits (especially Bananas) are fantastic for you and that the nutrients found in fruit and veg work wonders for our body in increasing energy, fighting disease and improving mental function.

But 5 fruits a day? That's quite a lot for most of us, right?

Unless you carry round a bunch of Bananas or a bag of apples and spend all day munching it can seem a little overwhelming to try and cram in 5 portions every single day.

But there is a way to cheat. A secret weapon:

Smoothies.

In case you've never come across them, smoothies are created by blending the flesh of a fruit, including all the pulp, sometimes excluding the skin, and creating a drink with a slightly thicker consistency than a juice.

The fantastic thing about them is that they can be made from all sorts of combinations including; Strawberries, Bananas, Passion Fruit, Mango, Orange and pretty much any delicious far flung fruit you can think of. They are easy to find in any supermarket and relatively cheap.

Heck, you can even make your own!

With that many fruits pressed and preserved into a single drink the nutritional benefits make smoothies one of the healthiest things you can drink. Typically a 250ml glass contains one or two of your 5-a-day fruit and veg needs.

Now let's imagine you had a single banana with your breakfast. (Excellent idea, right there. I wonder where you got that from?...) Then you have a quick smoothie drink before you start the work day. That's 3 of your 5-a-day already done!

Now you just need the other two which can be as simple as another glass later or including a small handful of vegetables in your lunch and dinner.

Bingo. We are at 5-a-day and it was easy and tasty!

If you do take up the smoothie route there are a couple of things to consider;

Smoothies vs. Juices

Both are great for you. Both offer essential amounts of vitamins C, naturally occurring sugars and both taste great, but in this case smoothies (usually) get the edge.

The difference presents in the way they are made.

Smoothies are made by blending the entire fruit, often including the skin, fiber and pulp while conversely juices extract just the water and nutrients and discard the rest.

Juices, being 'thinner' get nutrients into the blood stream quickly, which sounds like a good thing but it also means the fructose or fruit sugar, hits your body fast and causes the ups and downs of sugar spikes.

Smoothies however take a little longer to digest due to the extra content but because of this they provide a slower, more steady nutrient release, which prevents the blood sugar and mood spikes sometimes seen in sweet drinks. The body takes a little longer to process smoothies but it generates a flatter energy release while also providing much needed fiber which aids in digestion.

It's recommended to consume around 25g of fiber per day for women and 38grams for men. Smoothies help toward this while giving all the benefits of daily fruit intake.

Smoothies also tend to feel more filling because of the included fiber and so should be an essential part of your breakfast line-up. The best thing is that they are also so readily available. Yes, you can make your own but for most of us heading down to the supermarket and grabbing a couple of cartons is a quick and easy way to get more nutrients in our life.

Top Tip:

Look for *Fruit Only* smoothies. That means they only include the good stuff. Manufacturers are quick to call anything resembling fruit 'a smoothie' regardless of how many preservatives and junk additives are included. A favorite trick is also to include sugar in the ingredients.

A real smoothie shouldn't need it. Fruit is naturally sweet in most cases due to fructose and so if sugar or synthetic sugar is listed among the ingredients it is best avoided.

3. How to 'Top-Load' Your Day for Unstoppable Energy

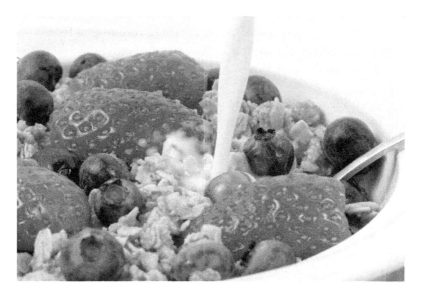

-*"Reverse your eating pattern for long-term energy."*

Another morning, another dash to the office, via dropping the kids at school/picking up lunch/putting fuel in the car/a million other things. Who has time for breakfast?

Answer: Everyone should.

Skipping breakfast is pretty much a mortal sin in terms of healthy eating and the idea of skipping breakfast to burn more calories is backwards logic since it actually causes over-eating later in the day. The truth is that breakfast can help you lose weight!

Overnight during sleep we go through 7-10 hours (hopefully) of fasting – hence the name, and we take on no fluids to hydrate the body. The first couple of hours after waking up are the time when your body most needs its food and drink.

But even of those of us that do grab breakfast 99% probably get it the wrong way around.

It's sometimes called the pyramid theory. IE We have a light breakfast, if any, a moderate lunch and then fill up on a large satisfying meal in the evening when we get home. We start with a small amount of food and our meals get bigger and heavier throughout the day.

But studies have shown this is literally an upside down way of doing it. Think about it, when do you most need your energy from food? During the day. So when do you least need it? In the evening prior to sleep.

So why are we all befuddled with our eating habits? A lot of it is simply tradition.

In the same way we usually serve food in the "Russian Style"; Service à la Russe - sequentially, with the starter, then main, then dessert, it has become customary for us barely eat in the morning and to load ourselves up with the heaviest and hardest to digest food last thing in the day.

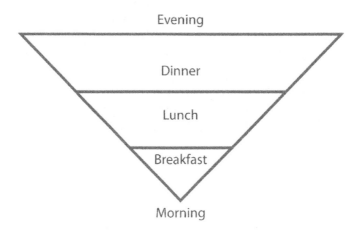

Can you see how unstable that looks?

Instead try flipping it around for all-day energy.

- Try Breakfast as a larger, hearty meal including perhaps Oats in the form of Porridge (High in Beta Glucans), a chopped Banana, a slice of wholemeal toast (Steady energy instead of spikes like white bread) and a glass of juice or fruit smoothie. Throw in a cup of tea or coffee if you don't overdo the sugar!

- Lunch, a moderate sized meal to sustain energy.

- Dinner, a lighter but still tasty meal. Perhaps soup or small dish.

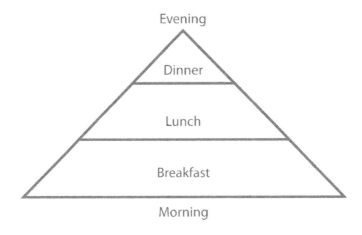

Note how much more stable the diagram now appears. Just like building a house a good breakfast foundation lays the ground work for your days' nutritional requirements and provides all day energy if done correctly.

The other way around provides energy when you need it least, which can even interfere with sleep.

Try the following motto:

"Breakfast like a King, Lunch like a Prince, Dinner like a pauper."

4. When to Fuel Up Before Your Workout

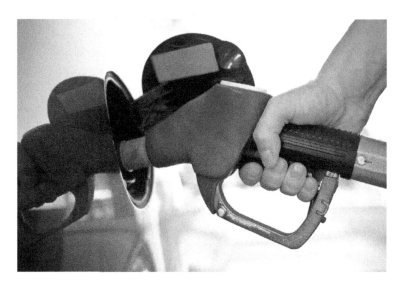

- *"Time your eating before your workout for optimal performance"*

When it comes to fueling up your workout, timing is everything. You should not eat immediately before your workout, but you also should not be active on an empty stomach either. This is especially true if you plan to workout for at least thirty minutes.

To get the maximum return from your food you should eat a snack between 45 minutes and 1 hour before your planned session, consume small meals around 1.5 to 2 hours before and large/normal meals around 3 hours before exercise. The closer it is to your workout time, the smaller your meal should be.

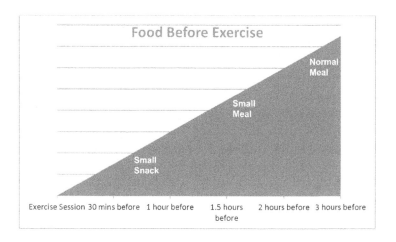

Food Before Exercise

Normal Meal

Small Meal

Small Snack

Exercise Session   30 mins before   1 hour before   1.5 hours before   2 hours before   3 hours before

Of course a small meal for one person may huge compared to another. For this reason you can use your own hands as a measuring guide. Hands are excellent since they are uniquely adapted for your own body size.

-   **Small snack = a fist-sized amount**
-   **Small meal = two fist sized amounts**
-   **Large Normal meal = 2 hands worth (or more)**

As a simple measuring device this is a good rule of thumb. Thumb, hands…get it? Sorry.

You might find that you feel better when you eat carbohydrates before your workout. Choose lower calorie carbohydrate rich foods with a bit of protein. Good options include vegetable slices and hummus, oatmeal, fruit, milk and cereal, toast with peanut butter, or a yogurt parfait. Listen to your body and you will learn what works best for you.

Regardless of what you choose, enjoy it with plenty of water. In fact, you should drink water throughout the day whether you plan to workout or not. Sports drinks are big right now, but you should save those for during or after your workout. If your planned session will be less than one hour then you really will not need these at all.

You may have heard that you will make your body burn fat when you exercise on an empty stomach. This is true, but it will not necessarily lead to overall body fat loss. As your glycogen, or carbohydrate, stores drop, your mental and physical functioning will suffer. Once your body begins to burn fat stores, you may feel your energy begin to sag. Your intensity will be lower, and you might run out of steam long before you meant for your workout to be over. As a result you will burn far fewer calories both per-minute and overall. Your body will burn more calories if you are in the carbohydrate-burning zone. You will also feel better both physically and emotionally. You will feel stronger and perform better so plan ahead and fuel up in advance.

5. Take Emotional Eating to the Curb

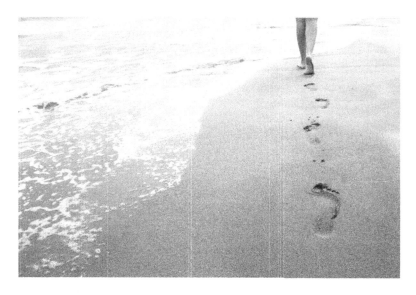

- *"Beat stress-eating with a walk"*

One of the best things you can do to safeguard your fitness goals is to banish emotional eating – one of the most common causes of poor diet choice. An easy way to do this is recognizing when your cravings are being brought on by stress then instead of eating, get outside and just take a walk. The fresh air will help you breath deep, and focus your mind.

Stress eating is extremely common. Even a small binge, around 200 calories for example, can make a difference on your waistline. If stress encourages you to eat just two of these extra snack a week, that adds up to 20,800 calories or 6 pounds across the span of a year. Consider the effects of keeping this bad habit for ten years and that adds up to an extra 60 pounds to burn (or carry!). More frightening is the thought that this is only a conservative estimate since most of us make very poor food choices when we are stressed.

By trading that snack for a short walk, you can eliminate at least 27 pounds across those same ten years. Next time you find yourself feeling stressed, close the refrigerator or cupboard door. Ask yourself if you are truly hungry, or trying to drown out a negative emotion. If the latter is your answer, then turn around and grab your shoes instead. Take a short, mindful walk. In addition to burning calories, you will get those feel-good endorphins pumping. You will feel better about yourself, burn a few calories, and get the stress break you needed in the first place. Do not let stress eating sabotage an otherwise healthy diet and lifestyle.

6. Organize Your Refrigerator

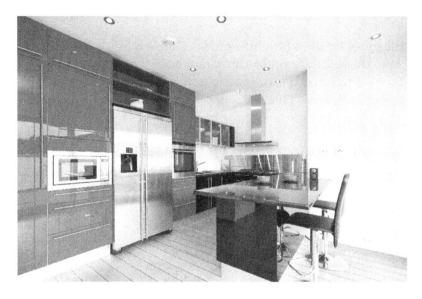

-   *"Stack up your fridge to encourage healthy choices"*

A little organization of your refrigerator has been proven to go a long way in regards to making healthier food choices. It will also make it easier to choose good foods over more junky varieties.

This tip will ensure that you make better choices throughout the week. So clear a small space in your schedule for cleaning, sorting, strategizing, and prep work, perhaps after you return from shopping at some point.

Research shows that people tend to choose from the middle of a fridge. Marketers have long known that the products in the middle shelves at the store receive the most attention. It works inside your own refrigerator as well. This is where your eyes focus first. Place your healthiest options on the center shelf.

Go a step further with a little prep work. Wash, peel, and slice vegetable sticks. Divide fruits, cheeses, and other healthy snacks in to reasonable portion sizes that are easy to grab and go. This will really help when you are in a hurry, or just too tired to put much effort.

If your fridge tends to be a little crowded, post a list of your options on the door after each shopping trip. Counteract the space war by cleaning out your refrigerator at least once a month. Toss anything that is expired or undesired. This will reduce your risk of food contamination as well as open up more space for fresh produce, and lean proteins.

The front of the fridge is highly visible but also typically the warmest with most exposure to the outside while the door opens, whereas the rear is the coolest.

Fridge Layout Principles:

Middle: Healthy foods

Lower (and out of sight): Unhealthy and junk food

Front: Healthy food that will not go off easily

Rear: Food that needs to remain cooler

After highlighting your best choices, work towards hiding less healthy indulgences out of sight. If you see an enticing food the moment you open the door, you become almost seventy percent more likely to choose it. Purchase opaque containers for storing your more sinful foods. By keeping the chocolate and other goodies out of sight, your attention will be drawn to better options. However, it will still be there when you are ready to seek out a treat. Just remember to enjoy your treat in moderation.

7. Brilliant Beta Glucans

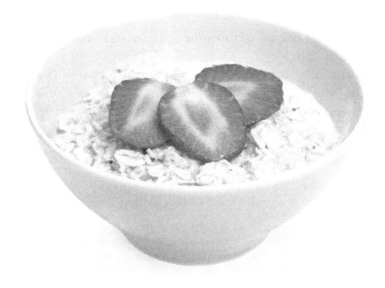

- *"Get some Beta Glucans in your diet for weight management, steady energy release and boosts to your immune system!"*

There are a million and one vitamins, minerals and nutrients currently claimed to have miraculous benefits to the human body but most fall apart, or at the very least are proven to do nothing, when examined under close scrutiny by the scientific community.

But one special type of fiber is consistently proving to be truly super among the super foods.

Beta-Glucans are a type of soluble fiber typically found in oats that studies are showing can have a range of excellent health benefits on the human body including lowering cholesterol, fighting disease and combatting allergies.

The European Journal of Nutrition even published recent findings that Beta Glucans of certain types prevent colds, reduce symptoms and even increase resistance to infections!

Studied benefits include:

- **Potential boosts to immune system and even combatting tumor cells (Journal of Immunology, European Journal of Nutrition)**
- **Fighting Seasonal Infections**
- **Combatting Allergies**
- **Lowering Cholesterol**
- **Longer 'full' feeling and reduced appetite**

If you are thinking this all sounds great you may be wondering how you get some of this wonder-stuff into your diet. Thankfully this is very easy.

Oatmeal or porridge oats is typically packed with Beta Glucans and since we already know that breakfast is a crucial meal in the day you can try introducing some porridge as part of your first meal of the day. A chopped Banana or other fruit can top it off and add some zest to the flavor.

8. Choosing Superfoods

Here's one of the most popular diet tips; *Eat more superfoods*

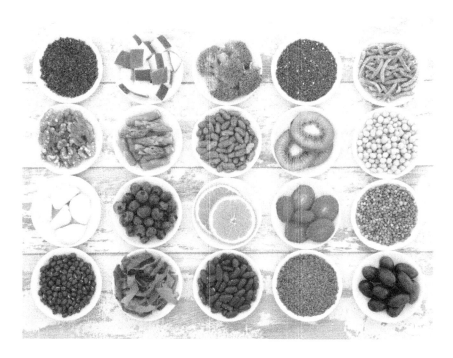

- *"Introducing superfoods can help your diet, but don't always believe the hype"*

Great, but what are superfoods?

If you believe the food aisles, 'superfoods' are pretty much anything considered slightly healthy that the manufacturers wish to sell quickly.

Garlic? Superfood!
Raspberries? Superfood!
Pizza...ok, maybe not.

In any case the concept of superfood has sadly exploded over recent years and has been exploited by sellers worldwide, leading to much confusion among the consumer. Not least because many food manufacturers fund their own highly weighted 'scientific' studies which miraculously espouse the benefits of the product in question.

The biggest issue lies in the way such testing is carried out. The extraction of chemicals and compounds within these food tests is undertaken in a way that would never occur in the body.

For example; Garlic was recently claimed to be a superfood because it reduces blood pressure and cholesterol diminishing chances of heart disease. This is true…if you eat the equivalent of 28 cloves a day, to match the samples used in the lab.

Superfoods are good for you, no doubt, but as part of a balanced diet already low in fatty, sugary foods.

The following is a list of common superfoods and a little balanced evidence for each to help you decide:

Popular Superfoods

1. Beetroot

Beetroot has been used medicinally for hundreds of years. Historic healers used beetroot to treat a variety of complaints such as constipation, fever, and skin disorders. Modern natural health practitioners continue to believe that beetroot can reduce your blood pressure, enhance your athletic abilities, and slow the progression of dementia.

Eating beetroot will provide your body with iron, folate, nitrates, magnesium, and a variety of antioxidants. Science suggests that your body will transform the nitrates into a chemical known as nitric oxide. This chemical has been linked with reduced blood pressure. A 2013 study with beetroot juice observed a slight lowering of blood pressure.

A second 2013 study focused on beetroot juice and enhanced athletic performance. The results showed that both sedentary and active participants received moderate increases in their ability to perform physical activities after incorporating beetroot juice into their diets.

An earlier experiment from 2010 looked at the relationship between beetroot juice and the slowed progression of dementia. While not entirely conclusive on the subject, this study did discover a possible increase in blood flow towards particular areas of the brain.

The Final Word:
Beetroot juice is a healthy choice. When incorporated into a well-balanced diet, the nitrates supplied by beetroot juice may reduce your blood pressure.

2. Blueberries

The blueberry is often praised for its antioxidant content. Some even boast its ability to prevent heart disease and cancer while boosting your memory. A closer look is required to determine the validity of these claims.

It is true that blueberries offer vitamin K, manganese, vitamin C, fiber, and a host of antioxidants including anthocyanin and phenolic compounds.

Research conducted in 2012 explored the connection between berry consumption and heart attack prevention. Some of the 93,000 women consumed at least three serving of strawberries and blueberries every week.

This group was compared to one in which the women only one serving of berries a month. The study found that the women who consumed three or more servings of berries every week exhibited a 32% reduced risk of heart attack.

In another interesting study, lab animals were fed blueberry extracts. These animals demonstrated reduced free radical damage. While this information might be useful in the prevention of cancer, it is unknown whether the human body would utilize the compounds in the same manner.

Some small-scale investigations also show a connection between eating blueberries and improved learning and memory skills.

The Final Word:

The research suggests that blueberries are a wise option for one of your daily fruit servings. Add them to cereal or yogurt for a morning treat.

3. Broccoli

Dark green vegetables, like broccoli, are often said to reduce your risk of many types of cancers including those of the stomach, mouth, and throat. In 2007 the World Cancer Research Fund conducted a close review of the information connecting broccoli to cancer prevention. In their conclusion they explained that, while it is possible that broccoli contains health-boosting compounds, further research is needed to validate such claims.

Research conducted in 2008 also looked at the effects the direct application of sulforaphane, an antioxidant found in broccoli, on human blood vessels. The sulforaphane seemed to protect the blood vessels against the damage associated with high blood sugar. However, the results were not conclusive enough to determine whether the antioxidant would effectively protect a diabetic from such damage.

In 2012, researchers looked at the potential benefits of broccoli consumption among 81 diabetics. The participants consumed 10 grams of enriched broccoli sprout powder once a day for a duration of four weeks. At the close of the study, researchers observed reduced cholesterol and triglyceride levels among the participants. Cholesterol and triglycerides are culprits in heart disease.

The Final Word:
While not all of the broccoli-related health claims can be substantiated, it is still a good source of many nutrients including vitamins a and c, fiber, folate, and calcium. These are essential for several of your body's functions. Try adding broccoli to your favorite soup, salad, or stir fry.

4. Chocolate

Chocolate fell into a whole new light when researchers, visiting Central America, stumbled upon the Kuna Indians in Panama. These people, who relied on cocoa as their primary drink, exhibited surprisingly low blood pressure levels. In response to this new information, some of the world's biggest chocolate manufacturers began boasting of the benefits of this superfood. Today it is believed that the antioxidants present in dark chocolate can relieve your stress and prevent cancer.

The cocoa used to prepare the beverages enjoyed by the Kuna Indians is similar to the cocoa which is used to produce chocolate. This cocoa contains many nutrients including iron, zinc, magnesium, phosphorus, and manganese. Additionally, it also provides two important antioxidants known as procyanidins and catechins.

In 2012, all of the respected evidence linking chocolate to reduced blood pressure was evaluated. A handful of the studies reviewed did support the idea that the consumption of cocoa could prevent cancer of the bowels.

Researchers took a look at the connection between chocolate and stress reduction in a 2009 investigation. In that study, 30 participants consumed 40 grams of dark chocolate every day for two weeks. While the final evaluation did show reduced stress hormone levels, the results must be weighed against the fact that the study was funded by a popular chocolate producer.

The Final Word:
It is difficult to assess the validity of the health claims associated with chocolate. Much of the research makes use of pure cocoa extracts, not candy bars. Even if the claims are true, you should save chocolate for a special treat. Most of the chocolate products at your local market will contain significant amounts of fat and sugar, which can spoil an otherwise healthy diet.

5. Garlic

If you scan the latest health magazines, you will see articles linking garlic to the prevention of high blood pressure, heart disease, high cholesterol, cancer, and even the common cold. While some of these claims are still pending approval, it is true that garlic provides some manganese, selenium, vitamin B6, and vitamin C. It also contains antioxidants such as allicin.

A 2012 review explored the findings of many respected studies which focused on the consumption of garlic and blood pressure reduction. One of those studies demonstrated that 200 milligrams of garlic ingested three times daily was effective in lowering blood pressure.

A separate review from 2009 took a closer look at 29 similar studies. Those studies seemed to show a slight reduction of cholesterol levels in the collective 1,794 participants with the consumption of garlic. While some studies also provide evidence that garlic consumption may reduce your risk of catching a cold, further research is needed.

Promising results resulted from the World Cancer Research Fund's 2007 review. They concluded that garlic could likely help to prevent cancers of the bowel and stomach. However, a similar review conducted in 2009 seemed to rule out the likelihood that garlic could prevent cancers of the breast, lung, or womb. That same review provides only a sliver of a hope that the superfood might reduce your risk of disease.

The Final Word:
It is clear that concentrated use of garlic can improve your cholesterol, circulation, and blood pressure levels. However, it is unknown whether a clove or two a day can provide significant results. Nonetheless, garlic is an excellent flavoring agent. For additional benefits, try using garlic in place of salt.

6. Goji Berries

Practitioners of traditional Chinese medicine have been using the goji berry for a span of over 6,000 years. Goji berries are said to boost your brain and immune system functions while preventing both cancer and heart disease. Some people even believe that goji berries can add years to your life. These signature red and wrinkled berries are a good source of vitamins A, B2, and C. They also provide iron, selenium, and a variety of antioxidants.

The British Diabetic Association has reviewed one of the more notorious studies involving goji berries. That trial discovered that ingesting 120 milliliters of goji berry juice every day for two weeks was enough to achieve a greater sense of well-being, better brain function, and improved digestion.

Another well-known study was conducted in China in 1994. That experiment involved 79 participants, who were all battling advanced forms of cancer. The group who were administered both immunotherapy and goji sourced polysaccharides, saw significant regression of their diseases. Still, some experts question the validity of this particular study.

The Final Word:
While some scientific trials have produced promising results, they have been conducted using concentrated and purified goji berry extracts. These extracts tend to be very expensive. While there is no harm in adding goji berries to your diet, you would be better off eating a wide variety of fruits and vegetables.

7. Green Tea

Practitioners of Chinese medicine have also been using green tea for hundreds of years. They often prescribe the tea for depression or headaches.

The way that green tea is processed is said to increase the saturation of antioxidants, making the compounds more concentrated than in other tea. You might have heard that green tea can be used to speed your metabolism, help you lose weight, reduce your cholesterol, treat or prevent heart disease, prevent cancer, and protect against Alzheimer's. While some of these claims may carry some truth, not all are accurate. It is true that green tea provides B vitamins, folate, magnesium, manganese, caffeine, potassium, and antioxidants. A specific group of antioxidants known as catechins, paired with the caffeine, do suggest that green tea could play a part in speeding your metabolism. This can lead to greater weight loss.

A 2010 investigation took a close look at 11 studies which focused on the connection between tea consumption and heart disease prevention. Amongst these studies there were 821 participants. Those who consumed black or green tea everyday showed reduced cholesterol and blood pressure levels. A second review from 2011 confirmed these findings. It seems conclusive that drinking green tea can reduce your risk of heart disease or stroke.

In 2010, a lab experiment looked at the effects of an enriched green tea extract on animal cells. The results showed that the tea provided protection against nerve death. Nerve death is one of the leading culprits in dementia and Alzheimer's. While promising, the effects have yet to be demonstrated with humans.

The Final Word:
Green tea is a great low-calorie beverage which can be safely enjoyed in moderation. While there is still much to learn about the benefits of drinking green tea, the research looks promising in regards to weight-loss and heart disease prevention.

8. Oily Fish

Researchers have discovered that the Eskimos, who rely on oily fish as their primary form of sustenance, experience significantly less heart attacks and strokes than similar populations. Since these observations were made, the oily fish has become attributed with a host of health claims. Sardines, salmon, and mackerel are said to help you avoid heart disease, cancer of the prostate, dementia, and vision loss.

If these claims prove to be true, they may be due in part to the concentrations of vitamin D, protein, selenium, omega-3 fatty acids, and the variety of B vitamins present in oily fish.

A 2004 declaration by the UK Scientific Advisory Committee on Nutrition states that the available research demonstrates that the consumption of oily fish can in fact reduce your risk of heart disease. The oily fish can reduce your blood pressure and remove dangerous fat clogs in your arteries.

While a 2012 review failed to find conclusive evidence that the omega-3 fatty acids found in oily fish can prevent dementia, there is still promising information that suggests the fish may slow macular degeneration. In both cases more research is needed before a final conclusion can be reached

The Final Word:
To receive the greatest benefits, you should consume at least two servings of fish every week. One of those portions should be of the oily fish variety. This should help reduce your blood pressure and reduce your overall risk of heart disease.

9. Pomegranate Juice

The pomegranate is a unique and easily-recognized fruit. There is no mistaking the bright red skin, or plump and delicate seeds. Medicinal preparations have made use of pomegranate for millennia. In the Middle East, pomegranate juice is thought to lower blood pressure, prevent heart disease, reduce inflammation, and prevent some forms of cancer, such as that of the prostate.

Some of these claims are supported by the nutritional content. Pomegranate provides you with vitamin C, fiber, vitamin E, iron, vitamins A, and a host of antioxidants.

A 2006 experiment, involving a small group of men, confirmed that a daily 8 ounce glass of pomegranate juice did slow the progression of prostate cancer. A shorter three month study in 2005 also saw improved circulation and a reduced heart attack risk in the participants who drank pomegranate juice.

Another study, which culminated in 2004, had its participants drink 1.7 ounces of pomegranate juice. The participants were carefully observed as they continued this pattern over the course of three years. During that time the cholesterol damage to their arteries improved by at least 50 percent.

The Final Word:
A small glass of pomegranate juice might be an enjoyable choice for one of your five daily fruits and vegetables. Opt for a bottle without any added sugar, or skip the juice and munch on whole pomegranate seeds.

10. Wheatgrass

In the 1930's an American Chemist known as Charles Schnabel inherited the nickname, "Mr. Wheatgrass". He ignited the fire of scientific interest in the potential health benefits of wheatgrass. Some health fanatics believe that wheatgrass is nutritionally superior to all other vegetables. Unfortunately, that claim appears to be little more than hype. Other claims suggest that wheatgrass may help increase your red blood cell count, prevent inflammation, and enhance your circulation.

In its defense, wheatgrass does provide vitamins A, C, and E, iron, magnesium, and calcium. However, the popular belief that a single shot of wheatgrass juice can provide a quantity of nutrients equal to that supplied by two pounds of vegetables does not stand up to the test. When evaluated pound for pound the nutritional content measures in line with standard vegetables like broccoli and spinach.

The idea that wheatgrass improves your red blood cell count stems from the belief that hemoglobin and chlorophyll are strikingly similar. While an interesting theory, this phenomenon has yet to be proven in a scientific trial.

However, a 2002 study did find that a group of participants, who suffered from ulcerative colitis, did see improvements over the course of one month. A 2004 investigation involving 32 participants with thalassemia also discovered that a group, who consumed 3.5 ounces of wheatgrass each day, required less blood transfusions over a 3 year period.

The Final Word:
Wheatgrass does carry some nutritional value, however one shot of wheatgrass does not make up an entire vegetable serving. If you enjoy wheatgrass, continue to add a shot to your favorite smoothie, just beware that it may not live up to the hype.

The takeaway from all this is that so-called 'superfoods' are nutritious and perhaps slightly more beneficial than most foods, but only as part of a normal balanced diet. Eating handfuls of Goji berries alone will not suddenly improve your body and each 'superfood' claim should be considered as part of a whole healthy diet.

9. The Great Vitamin Myth

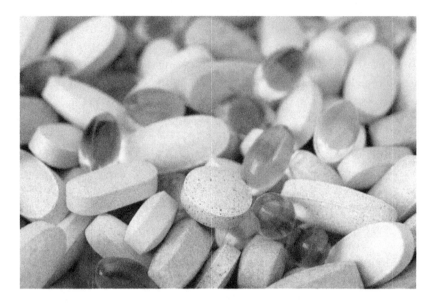

- *"Vitamin supplements may just be wasting your time and money!"*

If nutrition is a cash cow then the vitamin and supplements industry is an Everest-sized Aberdeen Angus.

The vitamin and supplement industry is worth billions of dollars worldwide and we guzzle down millions of pills every day. But do they actually do anything?

The manufacturers certainly think so, but then they would. There are also many scientific studies espousing the benefits of multi-vitamins but again many of these are funded, at least partially by the product makers, so results can be taken with a grain of salt.

Interestingly the latest impartial results seem to show that vitamin supplements aren't necessarily bad for us, they just aren't needed at all. A recent study carried out by the BBC and The University of East Anglia showed individuals typically received all of their nutritional requirements on a daily basis from their diet without any need from outside help. This was based on a very average diet with no special food or drink intake.

In fact individuals taking extra vitamin supplements were shown to simply pass the surplus straight into their urine.

Vitamins usually take two forms: Water Soluble types (Vit C and B) and fat soluble (A, and D etc). Bottom line is; if your body already has enough water soluble vitamins, and chances are unless you live in a deprived area it does, then you simply can't use any more. It goes straight into your pee.

The fat soluble vitamins are stored, unsurprisingly in body fat but also in the liver. Too many of these can actually be bad for you.

The FSA (Food Standards Agency) recently concluded that the average person gets everything they need from their diet and there are no 'boosts' to be had from overdoing it.

So are vitamins a waste of time? If you lead a normal lifestyle with an average balanced diet then yes, skip the vitamins and save the money. Or at least try it out and see how you feel.

But if you suffer from certain medical deficiencies or your doctor has suggested supplements then they definitely can help in these cases.

10. The Shocking Truth About Diets!

Here's an incredible fact you might not like to hear; dieting doesn't work and your body doesn't want it to!

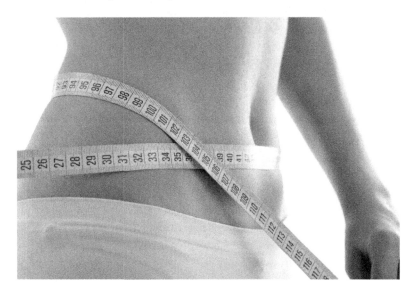

-   *"For real long term weight management avoid weight loss diets!"*

That's not to say you shouldn't have a healthy 'diet' in terms of regular meals. Your daily consumption of food is incredibly important and fuelling your body with the right stuff makes all the difference. But rapid weight-loss programs as a 'diet' have pretty much been categorically proven by the scientific community to fail.

It sounds counter-intuitive but the results show the best advice for long-term weight management is not to diet at all! – At least not in the way people think.

Diet in general refers to the food we consume every day but the idea of a restricted diet to control food intake is such a popular notion that an entire industry exists, worth millions of dollars each year.

The Paleo Diet, Atkins, South Beach; all are popular and all have famous celebrity advocates who claim that by eating like a caveman/tiger/lifeguard(?!) you can achieve your perfect body.

Yes they CAN work and the take-away word here is CAN. The models and uber-fit advocates you see for these systems probably did lose a lot of weight using these diets but the big difference, nay HUGE difference, is that it is short term weight loss is easy but the proven figures show around ninety percent of these people will pile the pounds back on within a year.

Research from Columbia University for example is one of many to show that once you lose weight quickly your body responds by switching on a mode of self-preservation that makes you actually burn less calories and feel more hungry – the complete opposite of what a dieter needs!

In fact their results showed that if you quickly lose say 50 pounds your body will now burn 20-25 percent less calories in activities and moderate exercise than someone who hadn't dieted at all. This of course makes it even harder to lose weight this way and only succeeds in depressing the dieter further, likely leading to binge eating and abandonment of the plan.

This vicious cycle destroys any hope of long term success.

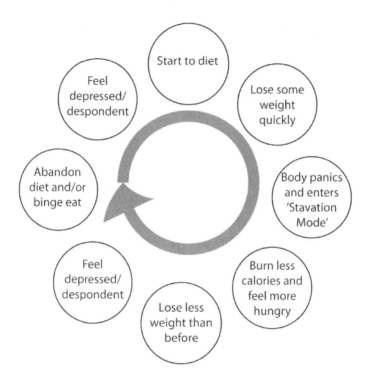

It's simply nature. This response evolved within us to ensure our species' survival during periods of very little food in pre-historic days. Today however we have the problem of obesity, an issue Mother Nature never accounted for.

The food you eat is absolutely crucial to improving fitness but trendy diets actually trigger a similar brain response to starvation.

An investigation by the University of Melbourne also found that hormones within overweight men and women went into overdrive once they started dieting. In particular Ghrelin – which stimulates appetite was higher, while Leptin – which suppresses it, was lower.

So how can we diet?

The trick in this case is not to throw your body into exotic and bizarre diets but to eat proper meals regularly and make small, manageable changes to the food you consume.

Lower fat and sugar intake while increasing protein and vegetables. It's really quite simple.

How to really keep the weight off:

Ninety percent of dieters failed within a year. So what did the successful ten percent do? They made realistic small changes and ate regular healthy food.

The National Weight Control Registry found that;

Of the successful dieters;

- Nearly 80 percent ate breakfast everyday
- Around 60 percent watched less than ten hours of TV per week
- Ninety percent performed moderate exercise for an hour each day – typically just walking.

So eat a good breakfast, switch off the TV and go for a walk once a day. Quick, easy and far more fun than fad diets!

Mind Hacks:

Mental motivation is the main driving force for fitness. If the body is the vehicle then the mind is the driver and if you can trick, fool or otherwise coerce the brain into enjoying exercise or improving diet you will find it much easier to create and stick to a schedule.

Best of all regular exercise has been proven to relieve stress and even treat mild to moderate depression, so a fitness routine is a healthy cycle that promotes both physical and mental wellbeing.

Of course our brain is also the most complex part of the body and takes a more subtle approach to manipulate, but get it right and you will have the most powerful tool in your fitness arsenal working for you.

The following tips focus on mental changes you can make in your daily lifestyle that will ultimately improve motivation and help you establish a healthy routine and happier existence.

1. Calendar Crosses for Unbeatable Habits

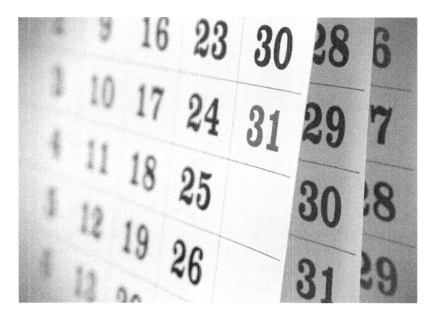

-   *"Mark your calendar each day for a motivation lift"*

A deceptively simple technique and one that I've mentioned in a couple of my books is the method of 'Calendar Crosses' for motivation.

Visual aids are for more effective for motivation that just willpower alone and Calendar Crosses make use of this principle to create a continuous run of workout days that you will wish to maintain.

If you've ever seen those movies where a prisoner scratches a mark on the wall for each day he has been incarcerated then the principle is similar only this time the system works in a positive way!

-   First you will need a large traditional calendar, the kind with a small box space for writing within each day.

- Place the calendar in a highly visible space. Perhaps where other family members or friends might see it

- Set your realistic but challenging fitness goal – say 10 minutes of exercise 5 days a week.

- Then draw a large visible cross in the box for that day on your calendar once you complete that goal.

(It can be a cross, mark or colored in box depending on your preference).

- Each and every day you complete your set exercise or task you add a mark to the box.

After a few days a colored shape starts to form on the calendar. Each block that you have marked adds to the pattern and reminds you how well you have done. If you have been coloring in the month notice how a solid block of color is forming.

Now, don't break the pattern.

Subconsciously we like consistency so you will be encouraged to maintain this pattern. A gap or white spot on an otherwise colored calendar will not only be an annoyance but a glaring sign to you and others that you skipped that day and did not complete your goal.

Top Tip:

If you are digitally minded there are phone applications that replicate this process. I personally find coloring in the squares physically cathartic but Apps like 'Commit' create a similar visual pattern for you to establish on your screen each time you confirm you completed an action.

2. The Right Words For You

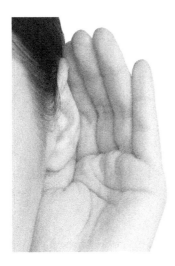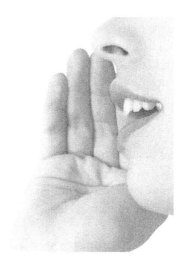

- *"The way you communicate has a big influence on your attitude to fitness, choose the right words!"*

Have you ever noticed the difference between top performers and those that just complain about wanting to be fitter or healthier? Of course you can spot the difference physically but you can also see how they differ in the way they present their thoughts through speech and writing.

It's a subtle difference but one that makes a big change. I call it the difference between 'do-ers' and 'say-ers'.

Most people will have great intentions of attending the gym, for example and say things like; *"I should really hit the gym more"* or *"I'm going to try and work out more often"* but then they don't. Why? Because they are already using negative, uncertain words.

But those who actually do get active will say things like *"I'm hitting the gym tonight"* or *"I'm getting in better shape this month"*.

Notice the change between the two? While one talks about their intentions then qualifies it with 'maybes' and 'Ifs' the other speaks with certainty as if there is no alternative. And psychologically for them there isn't, which is why they get it done.

We all know the things we need to do to get fitter but often we create mental friction by building these tasks up as a negative. We even build that negative in the manner in which we talk about them and when we finally add a "should" or "try" to the phrase it is basically like erecting a huge psychological barrier to the process.

These qualifying words create an obstacle and reinforce the concept that what we need to do will be hard work or unpleasant, despite the fact that it will be beneficial. As soon as we start throwing these terms around we may as well admit defeat.

Instead discuss what you will do as if there is no other option, as if it has already happened. This is not just for the benefit of those around you, who will now see you as a 'do-er' but for yourself. The simple act of saying "I'm hitting the gym tonight" is solidifying the idea in your mind.

There is no other option. It's already done.

You'll feel great for doing it and of course the fitness benefits speak for themselves.

It's not just speaking either. When you email or text a friend use the same language. No 'should' or 'try' but 'I will' or 'I am'. You are making a promise to yourself and those around you that you will be completing the task and they will respect you more for it.

Try it now!

In fact you can do it right now.

Leave a review for this book and in the comment tell everyone what you **WILL** do to improve your fitness. It doesn't have to be a huge change of lifestyle; even just a few tricks from this book can help, but make that statement about what is going to happen to improve your body now.

Top Tip:

To boost this process add specifics to your statements. "I'm going running twice this week" or "I'm making healthier dinner tonight". The specifics re-enforce the idea in your brain and combined with positive wording make for solid, healthy habits that are easy to maintain.

3. How to Physically Improve Your Brain - Learn How to Meditate in just 2 Minutes!

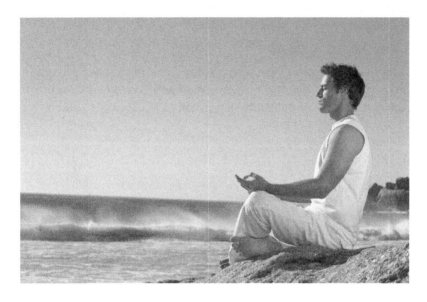

- *"Learn to meditate quickly and easily for proven physical and mental development"*

The benefits of Mediation are hard to overstate. In fact it's been proven that meditation helps your brain matter actually grow in beneficial ways.

But most people assume meditation requires achieving some kind of obscure inner enlightenment, moving to a mountain temple or hours of intense practice. All are untrue.

With even just 2 Minutes of Meditation per day you can improve focus, decrease stress and aid in your sleep. In fact researchers at Harvard Medical School discovered through the use of MRI scanning that Meditation directly affects the regions of the brain governing the autonomic nervous system. What this means to you is that by stimulating these parts of the brain we can expect to minimize stress, reduce blood pressure and improve digestion.

(This is a subject close to my heart and you can find out far more about techniques, benefits and Meditation tools in my book conveniently titled: *How to Meditate in Just 2 Minutes here:* http://bit.ly/1dYjnz6)

In the simplest form Meditation is just a calming of the body and centering of the thoughts. With this in mind there is no reason why you can't achieve this in just 2 minutes.

Meditation is always a personal experience and you are encouraged to approach it in whatever way is most comfortable to you. After reading through this guide you may find some techniques resonate more with you than others which is to be expected.

Once you have a preferred method you can incorporate this into your daily practice or regular schedule. But before you get to that point you may wish to begin with the most simple of the approaches: *2 Minute Breathing.*

Focused breathing forms the basis for the majority of all Meditation and Mindfulness exercises and so if you can perfect this you can easily move onto longer durations or other techniques.

The following breaks the process down into 30 second segments to further aid in structuring your approach. As always this is just a guide that can be modified as you see fit:

0-30 Seconds
- **Becoming Quiet and Still**

To start, your body and mind may be unsettled as you enter into the meditation. Use this first 30 seconds to do your best to become still and calm in both. Focus on staying in one position (of your choice) and slowing your thoughts. You may close your eyes to help this.

30-60 Seconds
- **Focus on the Breath**

Next, draw your attention to your breathing. Begin inhaling through your nose and out through your mouth. Focus fully on each breath and inhale for a mental count of 5, hold for a count of 2 and exhale for a count of 5. Then repeat.

60-90 Seconds
- **Expand Your Awareness**

Now allow your thoughts to expand and fully acknowledge your own body and all of its sensations. Don't judge or try to change anything. Allow your mind to be free of concern and become loosely aware of how that feels.

90-120 Seconds
- **Combine and Close**

With all the previous parts combined; stillness, focused breathing and a relaxed expanded awareness, you should find you feel calm and yet alert, focused and yet thought-free.

It is at this point where all the elements coalesce that you find the most power; a kind of therapeutic trance state which is almost impossible to put into words. (And feels completely unique for you so you don't need to try!)

Finally as the time draws to a close take some deeper breaths and draw your attention to the ground, chair or cushion on which you sit. Feel and listen for your physical surroundings and when you are ready open your eyes.

Don't Worry if it Doesn't Happen Right Away

The process above is the ideal way a brief 2 Minute meditation will play out but if it doesn't happen that way for you there is nothing to worry about.

It's very common for the process to be as different as the individual practising it. Simply use each 30 second strategy as a guide if you find your thoughts wandering, to bring them back in line.

Eventually you will find the process becomes second nature and you won't even need to think about it. The same approach can also be applied to longer sessions in the same way but for different durations.

Find out more in 'How to Meditate in Just 2 Minutes':
http://bit.ly/1dYjnz6

4. Why You Should Ditch Weigh-Ins and BMI B.S.

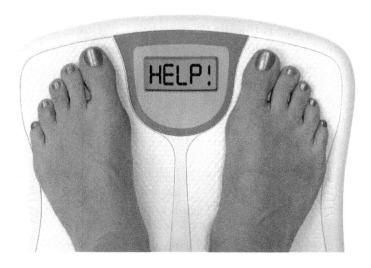

- *"Ditch the scales and BMI measurements and you are more likely to lose weight!"*

Do you dread the scales? Did you buy one of those fancy ones that electronically measures every facet of your body then depresses you with daily digital clarity?

You aren't alone. Most people have an unhealthy fear of finding out how much they weigh and when things appear to be going wrong they often abandon any healthy eating schemes thinking *"what's the point? It's not working anyway"*.

The truth is that your weight is only one of a number of measurements about your body, and not a very good one at that.

For starters your weight may not change (or may even increase) as you get fitter. Why? Because muscle weighs more than fat and all that tissue becoming toned will add to your total.

Additionally many experts now suggest that you should discard the scales altogether during fitness programmes as they offer more negative psychological barriers than benefits.

The human body is incredibly complex and fluctuations in weight occur all day, even after drinking something as simple as a glass of water. Seeing these in minute details can, for many people, be depressing or confusing leading to a downward psychological spiral.

So what about BMI – one of the most popular body composition measurements?

Nope, that can usually be ignored too.

The BMI (Body Mass Index) was created over a hundred years ago in the Nineteenth Century by a Belgian Polymath, (surely the sign of a fitness expert?!), as an early way to calculate an individual's fitness and body composition.

The formula is fairly simple: Your BMI is your mass in Kilos divided by your height in meters squared.

The astute among you will already see a problem here; it doesn't take into account the huge variability of humans as a species. A tall and big guy, even if incredibly muscular (since muscle weighs more than fat) will have a huge BMI score which would class him as dangerously overweight. In fact fitness barely comes into it.

A recent study by the BBC for example showed that many individuals scoring poorly on the BMI scale were actually 'fitter' than their "healthier" counterparts when tested running for a fixed period of time. Lung capacity, muscle condition, endurance and mental fortitude all make a big difference and none are measured using scales or the BMI process.

In fact most health authorities now acknowledge the limitations of BMI in measurement. The National Health Service for example says *"(BMI) itself is not a perfect measure of body fat and is not sensitive to the age-related changes in body fat distribution."*

And the National Heart, Lung and Blood Institute says; *"Although BMI can be used for most men and women, it does have some limits:*

- *It may overestimate body fat in athletes and others who have a muscular build.*

- *It may underestimate body fat in older persons and others who have lost muscle. "*

So what can I use?

Although fitness can be technically measured a number of ways (VO2 Max being the most popular) people usually don't have access to complicated equipment and treadmills for testing.

The easiest way to check if you are improving is to measure your recovery time from vigorous exercise.

How to measure your fitness:

1. Measure your resting pulse as beats per minute.
2. Now we aim to exercise (whatever type you want) to increase the resting rate to 60-80% of your maximum heartrate. (Maximum heartrate can be calculated as approximately 220 minus your age)

Age	Target Heartrate/Beats during Exercise
20–29	**120–160**
30–39	**114–152**
40–49	**108–144**
50–59	**102–136**
60–69	**96–128**
70–79	**90–120**

80–89	**84–112**
90–99	**78–104**
100 or older	**72–96**

3. Keep checking your pulse rate. (Monitoring devices like pulse-checking watches can help with this)
4. Once you hit the heartrate for your age as listed above stop completely.
5. Measure your heartrate immediately after stopping for a minute, then again 2 minutes after stopping.
6. Note down both the resting, immediate and 2 minute rates
7. The 2 minute figure minus the immediate figure gives a recovery rate. As you get fitter notice how this gets lower
8. Also notice how your pulse rate returns to the resting rate quicker as you improve.
9. Keep a note of these figures as your fitness increases

Aside from technically checking your pulse it should become obvious when you get fitter. Exercise becomes easier, chores are less exhausting and the idea of taking the stairs no longer fills you with dread!

So ditch the scales and arbitrary measurements. Fitness is about being active for yourself, doing the things that make you happy and enjoying life!

5. Turn Reps on Their Head to Make Exercise Easier

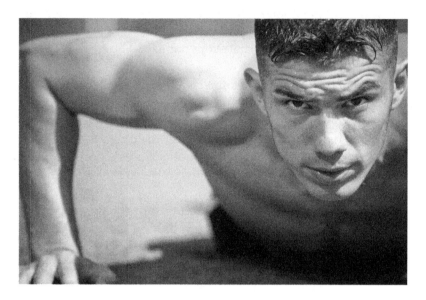

- *"Turn reps upside down to make exercise easier!"*

This is an old, but super-quick trick that instructors and fitness coaches have used for years. A. because we are sneaky sorts and B. because it works!

Anytime you complete a fixed number of reps (repetitions) for an exercise, drill or lift simply count backwards instead of up. Easy!

For example: nothing is more demoralizing than the idea of completing fifty push-ups. Beforehand we dread the idea and as you slog through them the numbers get higher and higher as the exercise gets harder and harder.

But switch it around and suddenly your brain is subconsciously imagining a lower number on each count, like a countdown to lift off. With each smaller number the set seems easier and the final goal closer, rather than further away as before.

So no more; "One, Two, Three, Four, god I hate my life – Five, Six.

Instead try; Six, Five Four, Three, Two, One. Done.

6. Hack Your Sleep, Recharge Your Mind (and Body)

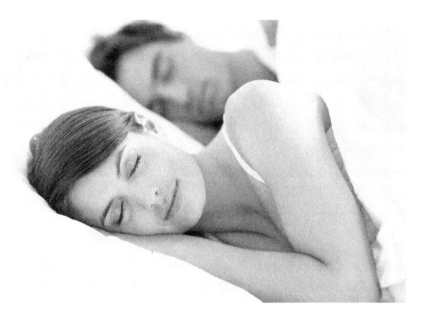

- *"Improve the quality (not necessarily quantity) of your sleep for a better body and mind!"*

Sleep is crucial but most people don't see its value for a fit, healthy body. Research, such as that performed by the University of British Columbia, has shown however that a reduction in sleep can have numerous negative psychological and physiological effects including raised blood pressure and reduction in bodily glucose control.

But indications are that better quality sleep is more important than pure quantity. A study in the Journal of Psychosomatic Research concluded that among the participants a good quality night's sleep was more effective than poor quality for a longer duration.

A few tricks and establishing a regular routine can ensure you get better quality downtime.

Sleep Tips (assuming you sleep at night):

- **Avoid caffeine after 5pm.**
- **Avoid eating after 8pm.**
- **Don't watch stimulating T.V, Movies, Games right before bed (Try reading).**
- **Make your sleeping location as dark as possible (Switch off led 'stand by' lights and try to block out street lights).**
- **Minimize noise when you sleep.**
- **Switch off or put away all your devices with glowing screens at least an hour before bed. (These confuse the brains Suprachiasmatic Nucleus into thinking it is day time)**
- **Exercise. (The National Sleep Foundation say that day time exercise improves evening sleep)**

The high-risk high-gain sleep hack

There is also an alternative, yet somewhat controversial trick whereby you can reduce your sleep time by hours, freeing up your day to be more productive than ever and still maintain your normal levels of functionality.

Is it worth it? I've personally never tried this tactic and I probably wouldn't, but those who do get it to work are very vocal about the benefits and let's face it, who wouldn't like an extra 5 hours in the day? Imagine what you could accomplish!

Polyphasic Sleep

While most people sleep utilize 'Monophasic sleep' for one long six to eight hour stretch per night Polyphasic sleep is a new concept involving sleeping for much shorter periods (20mins to four hours) many times during the day.

Studies show that shorter but more frequent naps within the Polyphasic approach actually trick the body into entering the most important, Stage 5 REM sleep segment, almost immediately. (Normally this can take up to an hour in traditional sleep patterns). Because the REM phase is so regenerative you can experience much less sleep but feel normal and operate successfully.

There are many approaches suggested for Polyphasic sleep and some are quite extreme but evidence suggests the most successful version, especially for beginners, employs one longer "core" sleep combined with several short naps throughout the day.

Example 1:

Over 24 hours
1x Core Sleep: 3 hours
3x 20 minute naps

Total: 4 Hours sleep
You gain: 4 Hours (Potentially)

Example 2:

Over 24 hours
1x Core Sleep: 1.5 hours
4x 20 minute naps

Total: 2.8 hours sleep
You gain: 5.2 hours (Potentially)

There isn't much more of a trick to it than that. Choose the time for your longer core nap, perhaps in the evening. Then throughout the day grab your short naps at regular intervals.

Note: The smaller core naps are crucial to this approach. If you are not in a position to be able to take short regular breaks (If you work in an office for example) then this technique is best avoided.

It's worth pointing out that while many people report great results and no health issues during Polyphasic sleep many others find it too difficult to adapt to. It is after all quite a change to your normal routine.

If you are thinking of introducing the technique try to do it at a time when your life is quite stable and you do not have important activities and work deadlines looming. If possible also tell a friend or relative what you are doing and ask that they keep track of your progress and monitor your health during the day.

7. Why You Should Forget Weight Loss (For Now)

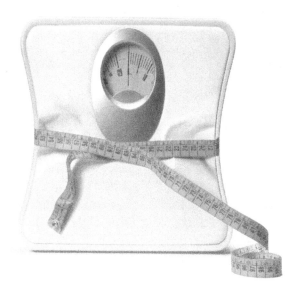

- *"Think of weight loss as a secondary goal to fitness and you are more likely to manage your weight successfully!"*

Most people have a love/hate relationship with weight loss. Love the idea, hate the process. Yes, lots of us would like to shed a few pounds but purely focusing on weight loss has been shown to make the actual process of losing weight more difficult, especially early on.

The mindset in which you approach weight loss is crucial and too many people see the numbers on a scale as the gospel. The problem with this is that initially weight loss is a slow process. Most people don't suddenly drop pounds overnight and in fact as a sustainable lifestyle change they shouldn't.

After all the human body is the master of adapting, as we've already mentioned, and once you cut out a huge portion of calorific intake the body slows down its usage to better preserve the condition it is in.

This of course means many people get despondent about early weight loss and give up. Instead consider this mantra:

"Fitness First"

The reality is that fitness and weight loss lead a symbiotic relationship. Introducing a more active lifestyle is a far more healthy approach to long term improvements. Find those spots where you can include a little exercise and establish a routine. ***Ignore the scales – don't get caught in the numbers game.***

I personally recommend only a single weight check and then no more for at least a month. During this month you establish your new fitter paradigm. Go for small manageable changes (like the tips included in this book) and make sure you stick to them.

Once you have a more active routine in place the fat will be dropping but muscle may be increasing. This could mean that weight doesn't drop much – but who cares! You will be fitter, healthier and look better than ever before and your new lifestyle is with you for the rest of your life. The numbers on a scale are just that, numbers, and they have little bearing on how you live your life.

Forget 'weight loss' and focus on just being fitter. In no-time at all you will find the weight falling anyway. Slow, steady progress and small easy changes are the key to a long-lasting healthy body.

8. Run...for Survival!

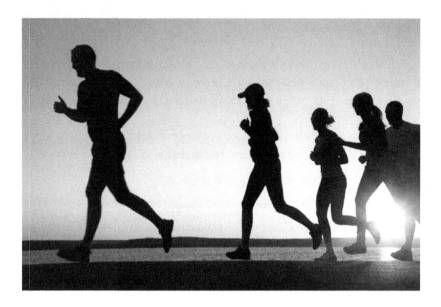

- *"Use fun Apps to turn running into a game!"*

The undead have risen and if you don't get moving they will eat your brains!

Rule no.1 in escaping the zombies: Cardio.

At least that's the type of plot behind "Zombies, Run!" and a number of other fun applications available for modern cell phones that track your running habits and generate a game as you move.

There are a series of apps available that take this approach, turning your regular exercise session into a battle against zombies, imaginary athletes or other runners. These clever programs use your phone's in-built GPS to track your progress and generate a game based on set parameters and your previous runs then give you feedback appropriately.

If you focus on the game they can generate fun feelings of competition, survival and camaraderie - all triggering primal motivation centers of the brain.

The great part of apps like this is that they also distract our mind from the hard work and engage a competitive part of us which makes us work harder. It is a similar principle to working out with a friend only this competition is with yourself and the undead of course.

9. Live In the Now and Destroy Mental Resistance

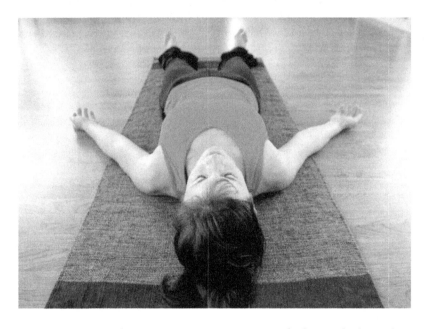

- *"Focus on the present to remove psychological obstacles!"*

As we've previously discussed one of the biggest obstacles to motivation in fitness is the mental resistance we manufacture ourselves. We've already covered several techniques for smoothing out this brain friction but one technique that consistently proves successful is to bring our focus into the moment.

Because we live in such information heavy times we are constantly planning and plotting and reviewing every event in our lives. This can be good in organizing our lives and getting things done but it does lead to thoughts weighing heavy on our conscience during the day.

As the day bears on the idea of your workout becomes more and more tiresome. Of course a simple approach is to get your workouts completed early in the day each time, as we've already mentioned in this book but another method you can use is a visualization exercise; 'Mental Filing'.

Mental filing is based around being in the present. At its core it is focusing on how you feel right there and then not what is to come or what has been but the present.

In an office environment once something is filed away it is safe, secure, out of sight and can be forgotten about until it is needed. This is the principle you will apply to thoughts of your gym session or workout.

Mental Filing:

- First thing in the day mentally run through what needs to be done

- Once you acknowledge the fitness activities you need to complete imagine writing them on a piece of paper and putting it away in a daily filing cabinet. Really try to visualize the details of this storages unit, its height, size and feel.

- During the day try not to think about the activity, knowing only that it is safely filed away and will be completed later.

- Any time your mind drifts back to the dreaded thought of attending the gym or completing that workout try to imagine taking that thought on the paper and placing it back into the filing cabinet, closing the door and walking away.

- Sure the door may occasionally pop open, and that's ok, but once the thought is safely inside you only need to retrieve it right before you begin the activity.

At the end of each day you can clear out the contents and get ready for the next. Always aware of what you need to complete but not thinking about it or building unnecessary resistance.

10. The One Incredible Thing You Can Do Right Now to Feel Instantly Happier

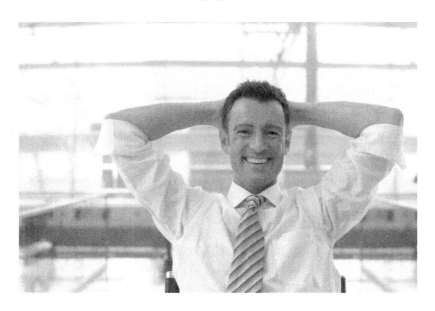

- *"Just smile!"*

If you're as cynical as me you see headlines like this and start to groan, but incredibly science has once again shown that the human body can be controlled far more than we think and that happiness can in fact be hacked.

I wanted to leave you with one final trick that can have you feeling better, even if nothing else has worked. Best of all it takes seconds.

Most people partake in fitness to feel happier. Happier about their body, their health and their mood.

Of course we all want to be more happy generally but feeling more upbeat is also proven to have positive benefits in all aspects of your life; including fitness. After all if you are happier you are more likely to feel good about staying in shape and so the positive reinforcement continues.

If you need a quick boost however here is one tip:

Smile (Even if you don't mean it). Experiencing a simple smile, whether first or second hand has been proven in numerous experiments to make you feel happier.

An Anchorage University study carried out for the Journal of Personality and Social Psychology discovered that just making a "Smiling Face" was sufficient to increase positive mood in participants. Equally other studies have found that simple exposure to a smiling expression raises mood.

Instinctively we are still programmed to associate a happy face with happiness, even if fake, so experiencing one yourself or on others starts to immediately brighten our outlook.

For increased effectiveness it was also found that self-exposure to the smile through use of a mirror made the trick more powerful and improved demeanour even more. Up to double the effect in fact.

However the opposite was also shown to be true so take care. Frowning and sad faces decreased mood even in cases where the subject started out happy.

So get that mirror out and remember the old saying, "Smile and the whole world smiles with you"!

Bonus Quick Tips

Don't have time to read the previous tips? (What are you the president or something?) Not to worry, the following are extra quick tips and instant fixes proving that even in the information-rich world we live in you can learn something new about how to use your body every day.

1. Get started now; it's never too late

Think you are too old to start improving your health? Think again.

It's never too late to begin improving your health and reap the benefits. A 2009 Swedish study carried out on thousands of men showed that even becoming more active between 50 and 60 years old yielded improved health and longer lifespan similar to those that had exercised for years before.

2. The carrot works better than the stick

Positive reinforcement has been proven to work better in establishing beneficial habits that punishing yourself for not adhering to them. BF Skinner, famed Psychologist, found that focusing on adding something good to a scenario establishes a pattern far more successful than punishment or taking something away.

3. Exercise to beat stress

There are many, many studies demonstrating this. If you are feeling down getting the heart rate up a little can and will help. The British National Health Service for example lists exercise as an effective treatment for stress, depression and anxiety. In some cases just as effective as medication.

4. Sleep in your workout clothes

If you sleep in your T-shirt and jogging pants you will wake up and be completely ready for your morning run or workout without any fumbling around or choosing clothing. Best of all gym clothing is usually very comfortable!

5. Schedule, Schedule, Schedule

Planning is key to an effective fitness routine and especially important in establishing long-term healthy paradigms. Look at your daily routine realistically and find the gaps for your exercise then make these part of your calendar as much as visiting the Dentist or going to work.

Thank You (and a Free Book!)

We always get out what we put in throughout life and fitness is no exception. Train smart and look after your body and it will look after you for many years.

Thanks to all the scientists, researchers and people pushing forward our knowledge of the human body. Thanks to Derek Doepker for his always helpful insights and thanks especially to you for reading this book. I work hard to create useful and easy-to-follow guides for martial arts, fitness and well-being.

Please help other readers and give this book 5 stars and a quick review if you found it helpful!

Good reviews make a world of difference to authors and other readers alike.

Finally, for your **COMPLETELY FREE** book check out my site at:

www.BlackBeltFit.com

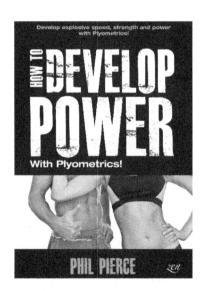

Thanks again.
- *Phil*

Other Books by Phil Pierce

Check out some of the other Martial Arts, Fitness and Well-Being titles from Phil Pierce:

How to Meditate in Just 2 Minutes: Easy Meditation for Beginners and Experts Alike

http://bit.ly/1dYjnz6

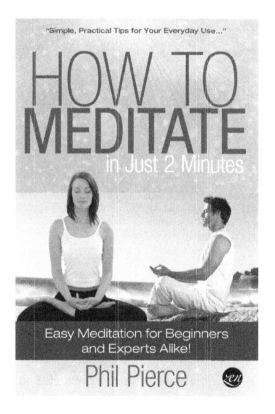

Given, Meditation can be an incredibly powerful tool in improving both physical and mental health, focus and relaxation but most people think it takes a long time to see results. The truth is, it doesn't!

With this easy-to-use book you can quickly learn how to achieve these incredible benefits in just 2 Minutes a day...

Bodyweight Training Handbook: Bodyweight Exercises, Tips & Tricks to Lose Weight, Build Muscle and Get Fit Fast!

http://bit.ly/1ncr5y2

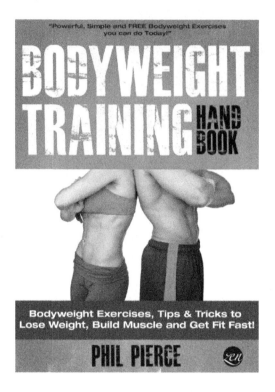

The #1 Fitness Bestseller - Grab Your Copy Now!

Discover the secrets the gyms don't want you to know...

How to get in amazing shape with top powerful, simple and free bodyweight exercises!

How to Defend Yourself in 3 Seconds (or Less): The Self Defense Secrets You Need to Know!

http://bit.ly/HdYSDE

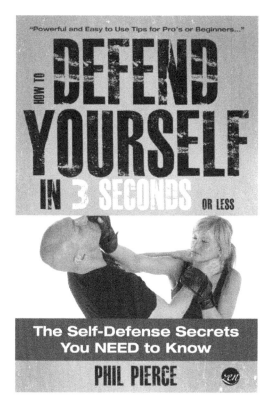

With most violent encounters the ability to defend yourself comes down to a matter of seconds where the right actions can be the difference between life and death.

Developed with input from Top Martial Artists and Self Defense experts this illustrated guide reveals the secrets of real Self Defence and exposes the truth behind street violence.

All designed to give you straight-forward, practical advice and keep you safe when it counts...

Made in the USA
Las Vegas, NV
29 March 2023

69843144R00095